CHILD HEALTH CARE COMMUNICATIONS

Summary Publications in the Johnson & Johnson Baby Products Company Pediatric Round Table Series:

1. *Maternal Attachment and Mothering Disorders: A Round Table*
   Edited by Marshall H. Klaus, M.D.,
   	Treville Leger and
   	Mary Anne Trause, Ph.D.

2. *Social Responsiveness of Infants*
   Edited by Evelyn B. Thoman, Ph.D., and
   	Sharland Trotter

3. *Learning Through Play*
   By Paul Chance, Ph.D.

4. *The Communication Game*
   Edited by Abigail Peterson Reilly, Ph.D.

5. *Infants At Risk: Assessment and Intervention*
   Edited by Catherine Caldwell Brown

6. *Birth, Interaction and Attachment*
   Edited by Marshall Klaus, M.D. and
   	Martha Oschrin Robertson

7. *Minimizing High-Risk Parenting*
   Edited by Valerie J. Sasserath, Ph.D. and
   	Robert A. Hoekelman, M.D.

8. *Child Health Care Communications*
   Edited by Susan M. Thornton, M.S. and
   	William K. Frankenburg, M.D.

Cover: *William K. Frankenburg, M.D., uses a videotape of Andrew Selig, Sc.D., counseling a family to demonstrate a successful communication technique for professionals attending a seminar on child health care.*

Cover Photo: *Marlin Cohrs*

CHILD HEALTH CARE COMMUNICATIONS

Enhancing Interactions
Among Professionals,
Parents and Children

Edited by
Susan M. Thornton
and
William K. Frankenburg, M.D.

Foreword by
Morris Green, M.D.

Introduction by
William K. Frankenburg, M.D.

Sponsored by

Johnson & Johnson
BABY PRODUCTS COMPANY

Library of Congress Cataloging in Publication Data
Main entry under title:

Child health care communications

(Johnson & Johnson Baby Products Company pediatric round table; 8)

Bibliography: p.
1. Children—Care and hygiene—Addresses, essays, lectures. 2. Communication in pediatrics—Addresses, essays, lectures. 3. Interpersonal communication—Addresses, essays, lectures. 4. Parent and child—Addresses, essays, lectures. I. Thornton, Susan M. II. Frankenburg, William K. III. Johnson & Johnson Baby Products Company. IV. Series.

RJ101C519   1983   618.92   83-6105

ISBN 0-931562-08-2

Copyright © 1983 by Johnson & Johnson Baby Products Company.

Printed in the United States of America. All rights reserved. Except as permitted under the Copyright Act of 1976, no part of this publication may be reproduced or distributed in any form or by any means or stored in a data base or retrieval system, without the prior written permission of the publisher.

*For all who seek to enhance
communications in child health*

CONTENTS

List of Participants	ix
Preface Robert B. Rock, Jr., M.A., M.P.A.	xi
Foreword Morris Green, M.D.	xiii
Introduction William K. Frankenburg, M.D.	xvii

PART I—AREAS OF NEED FOR IMPROVED HEALTH CARE COMMUNICATIONS

Introduction Susan M. Thornton, M.S.	1
The Need for a Family Orientation Andrew L. Selig, M.S.W., Sc.D. and Ellen W. Selig, M.Ed.	5
The Need to Teach Self-Care Skills Lorna M. Facteau, R.N., M.S.	14
Doctor-Patient Communication in Acute Child Health Barbara M. Korsch, M.D.	19
The Development of Concepts About Illness Ellen C. Perrin, M.D.	32
Communicating with Children in the Hospital Robert H. Pantell, M.D. and Catherine C. Lewis, Ph.D.	41
The Child with a Chronic Illness Michael Weitzman, M.D.	52
The Parent's Perception: **Orientating Parents to Their Responsibility** Suzie Rimstidt	61
Parents' Groups and Their Role in **Effective Communication** Susan Kelley MacDonald, M.A.	69
Communication Issues: **The Child with a Developmental Disability** Jean K. Elder, Ph.D.	77
Communicating with Community-Based Care Providers Jon Ziarnik, Ph.D.	83
Well Child Care Robert W. Chamberlin, M.D., M.P.H.	89

PART II—STRATEGIES FOR TEACHING BETTER COMMUNICATION

Introduction — Susan M. Thornton, M.S. — 97

Enhancing Communication Among Children and Adults Who Care for Them — Charles E. Lewis, M.D., Sc.D. and Mary Ann Lewis, R.N., M.S. — 99

Training Nurses — Judith Bellaire Igoe, R.N., M.S. — 111

Goals, Roles, and Content of Parent-Professional Interaction: Parent Education and Parent Support — Earl S. Schaefer, Ph.D. — 120

Strategies for Training Physicians in Effective Interpersonal Communication Skills — J. Larry Hornsby, Ed.D. — 131

Child Health Care Communications: Preparing Physicians in Training — Evan Charney, M.D. — 141

PART III—TECHNIQUES FOR IMPLEMENTATION: CURRENT POSITION AND FUTURE OPPORTUNITIES

Introduction — Susan M. Thornton, M.S. — 153

Academic Training/Medical Education — August G. Swanson, M.D. — 155

Nursing Education — Joy Hinson Penticuff, R.N., Ph.D. — 162

Practicing Nurse Practitioners — Karen Fond, R.N., M.S.N. — 174

The Physician's Role as a Communicator in Child Health Care — James E. Strain, M.D. — 181

Public Policy to Promote Better Communication — Lisbeth Bamberger Schorr — 189

APPENDIX A—Communication Guidelines — 196

APPENDIX B—Selected Communications Examples — 199

Bibliography — 213

PARTICIPANTS

Robert W. Chamberlin, M.D., M.P.H.
Maternal Child Health Consultant —
  Billings Area
Indian Health Service
Billings, Montana 59103

Evan Charney, M.D.
Pediatrician-in-Chief
Department of Pediatrics
Sinai Hospital of Baltimore
Baltimore, Maryland 21215

James T. Dettre
Director of Marketing Services
Johnson & Johnson Baby Products
  Company
Skillman, New Jersey 08558

William C. Egan
Director of Product Management
Johnson & Johnson Baby Products
  Company
Skillman, New Jersey 08558

Jean K. Elder, Ph.D.
Commissioner, Administration on
  Developmental Disabilities
Department of Health and Human
  Services
Washington, D.C. 20201

Lorna M. Facteau, R.N., M.S.
Instructor, School of Nursing
The Catholic University of America
Washington, D.C. 22064

Karen Fond, R.N., M.S.N.
Immediate Past President, NAPNAP
Pediatric Nurse Practitioner
Division of Primary Care-Pediatrics
University of California, Los Angeles
Los Angeles, California 90024

William K. Frankenburg, M.D.
Professor of Pediatrics and
  Preventive Medicine
Director, Rocky Mountain Child
  Development Center
University of Colorado
  Health Sciences Center
School of Medicine
Denver, Colorado 80262

J. Larry Hornsby, Ed.D.
Associate Professor of Psychology
Director, Behavioral Medicine
Department of Family Practice
Medical College of Georgia
Augusta, Georgia 30912

Judith Bellaire Igoe, R.N., M.S.
Associate Professor
School of Nursing
Director, School Health Programs
University of Colorado
  Health Sciences Center
Denver, Colorado 80262

Barbara M. Korsch, M.D.
Head, Division of General Pediatrics
Children's Hospital of Los Angeles
Los Angeles, California 90027

Charles E. Lewis, M.D., Sc.D.
Department of Medicine
University of California, Los Angeles
School of Medicine
Los Angeles, California 90024

Mary Ann Lewis, R.N., M.S.
Adjunct Associate Professor of
  Nursing and Medicine
University of California, Los Angeles
Department of Medicine
Los Angeles, California 90024

Susan Kelley MacDonald, M.A.
Prescription Parents, Inc.
41 Longfellow Road
Watertown, Massachusetts 02172

Robert H. Pantell, M.D.
Associate Professor of Pediatrics
Director, Division of General
  Pediatrics
University of California,
  San Francisco
San Francisco, California 94143

Joy Hinson Penticuff, R.N., Ph.D.
Assistant Professor
School of Nursing
University of Texas at Austin
Austin, Texas 78701

Ellen C. Perrin, M.D.
Assistant Professor of Pediatrics
Department of Pediatrics
Vanderbilt University Medical
 Center
Nashville, Tennessee 37232

Bonnie J. Petrauskas
Professional Relations
Johnson & Johnson Baby Products
 Company
Skillman, New Jersey 08558

Suzie Rimstidt
516 Hamilton Court
Bloomington, Indiana 47401

Robert B. Rock, Jr., M.A., M.P.A.
Director of Professional Relations
Johnson & Johnson Baby Products
 Company
Skillman, New Jersey 08558

Steven Sawchuk, M.D.
Chairman, Institute for Pediatric
 Service
Director of Medical Services
Johnson & Johnson Baby Products
 Company
Skillman, New Jersey 08558

Earl S. Schaefer, Ph.D.
School of Public Health
Department of Maternal and
 Child Health
University of North Carolina
Chapel Hill, North Carolina 27514

Lisbeth Bamberger Schorr
Co-Director, Child Health Outcomes
 Project
University of North Carolina
3113 Woodley Road, N.W.
Washington, D.C. 20008

Andrew L. Selig, M.S.W., Sc.D.
Associate Professor of Psychiatry
Chief of Social Work
Rocky Mountain Child
 Development Center
University of Colorado
Health Sciences Center
School of Medicine
Denver, Colorado 80262

James E. Strain, M.D.
President, 1982-83, American
 Academy of Pediatrics
Clinical Professor of Pediatrics
University of Colorado
Health Sciences Center
Denver, Colorado 80262

August G. Swanson, M.D.
Director, Department of Academic
 Affairs
Association of American Medical
 Colleges
Washington, D.C. 20036

Susan M. Thornton, M.S.
Science Writer
474 W. Easter Avenue
Littleton, Colorado 80120

James R. Utaski
President, Johnson & Johnson
 Baby Products Company
Skillman, New Jersey 08558

Michael Weitzman, M.D.
Assistant Professor of Pediatrics
Boston University School of
 Medicine
Boston City Hospital
Boston, Massachusetts 02118

Jon Ziarnik, Ph.D.
Associate Director for
 Community Education
Rocky Mountain Child
 Development Center
University of Colorado Health
 Sciences Center
School of Medicine
Denver, Colorado 80262

PREFACE

During the course of previous Pediatric Round Table presentations, a particular concept was reiterated with increasing frequency. Participants acknowledged that they were among professionals who frequently did not communicate very well, either with other professionals or — more importantly — with their young patients and their parents. Out of this increasingly obvious need for improved communications came the decision to hold a Round Table devoted to the topic of child health care communications. The Johnson & Johnson Baby Products Company felt this subject was so important that they wanted to bring together leading authorities in the field to discuss communication issues and publish their findings. Moreover, the Company felt a strong desire to actively contribute to improving future prospects for these communications.

With the enthusiastic support of the Round Table's Moderator, William K. Frankenburg, M.D., Director of the Rocky Mountain Child Development Center at the University of Colorado School of Medicine in Denver, the participants in this discussion were given an added challenge. This was to develop communication guidelines which, it was hoped, could be acted upon by persons involved in the health care of children. Dr. Frankenburg emphasized that the Round Table's overall goal would be to facilitate change wherever possible.

The participants sparked to the challenge. They developed first a framework of assumptions, and then came to general consensus on a set of communication guidelines which broadly focuses on three concepts in child health care communication:

1. There should be explicit training of health professionals in communication skills at every level of training (medical school, residency, and continuing education); integration of this training with biomedical training; nurturing of physicians in training to enhance their capacity for supportive interpersonal interactions; and modeling of interpersonal skills from respected and valued mentors.
2. There should be financing and organization of health services delivery to permit and support the use of good communication skills.
3. There should be action by parents, patients, and groups of concerned citizens and professionals to bring about desired changes

in health institutions in the allocation of resources, in health legislation, and in administration of health programs.

The sample communication examples which follow the communication guidelines in this publication are selected from a publication which contains 36 such examples titled "Communications Examples for Child Health." These examples have been developed to help highlight some of the innovative efforts underway in this country to improve child health care communications. The examples are centered around clinical and teaching situations and have been ably edited and cross-referenced by Science Writer/Editor, Susan M. Thornton.

It is with most sincere appreciation that the Johnson & Johnson Baby Products Company congratulates the 24 child health care authorities who participated in achieving the extended contributions of this Round Table. The combined results of this summary publication, the communication guidelines, and the communications examples should prove to be highly effective teaching tools and thus should make a significant contribution to improving child health care for professionals, parents, and children. We, as a company which feels its first responsibility is to its customers (both professionals and consumers), are proud to be associated with this publication and with the authorities who have made it a reality.

Robert B. Rock, Jr., M.A., M.P.A.
Director of Professional Relations

FOREWORD

Communication, the preeminent requirement for any satisfying and productive personal or professional relationship, remains an imperfectly understood, regularly overestimated, generally unquestioned, insufficiently studied, and incompletely applied process. This Round Table is dedicated to the belief that improved communication between health professionals and patients can enhance child health status and family functioning by achieving decreased suffering, lower morbidity and mortality, reduced health costs, greater patient and family functioning, augmented health professional satisfaction and productivity, and improved coordination of services.

Although a considerable amount is known about the affective, cognitive, verbal, and nonverbal aspects of communication, the clinical application of this knowledge is highly dependent upon the personality and experience of health professionals and the expectations and background of patients. It is well known, for example, that:

1. Communication is facilitated if the professional is a warm, friendly, nonjudgmental, responsive, and courteous person who sincerely wishes to understand the patient's needs and who regularly explains his or her findings and recommendations.
2. Communication is enhanced by continuity in the professional-patient-family relationship.
3. Skillful interviewing which draws upon a large repertoire of ways of responding to or engaging in exchanges with the child and family and which is tailored to the individual child and family is a vital force in communication.
4. The highly personal character of clinical care takes into consideration the child's health status, developmental stage, level of cognitive development and history, and the family's functioning, socioeconomic circumstances, and belief systems and culture.
5. Each child and parent should feel the professional's interest, conveyed, in part, by a personal style that is characterized by genuineness and graciousness.
6. The effective clinician has a scientific curiosity about people and a highly developed ability to *see,* to *hear,* to *feel,* to *empathize,* and to *read* the patient. The child and parent need to believe that the professional understands their concerns, is aware of what they think is wrong, wants to know what they

have done about it, is interested in what they expect, and senses how they feel.
7. The patient's questions must be answered and his or her expectations dealt with in some manner. Ideally, the professional's and the patient's perception of the problem and what needs to be done are congruent, but when it is not — as so frequently is the case — the professional should understand what the patient is attempting to communicate.
8. The professional who is interested in promoting communication permits the child and the parents to discuss their strengths as well as their problems and takes the opportunity, present during each visit, to commend them in some way.
9. An important goal of communication is for the child — through the process of identification with the health professional — to adopt the clinician's attitudes toward children's health. This is enhanced by the professional who has the ability to elicit children's trust, to develop a comfortable and friendly atmosphere, and to relate to children in a strongly positive fashion.
10. Patients who feel positively evaluated are likely to accept the health professional's recommendations. Communication, cooperation, and satisfaction are positively correlated with the patient's *reflective self-concept,* the self-evaluation which a patient makes through the professional's eyes (for example, "He likes me," "She thinks I'm a good mother," or "He trusts me to follow his advice.").

Why are these self-evidence principles so underutilized?

One reason is that relatively little time in medical training is devoted to the affective aspects of professional-patient relationships and to interpersonal communication skills on a day-to-day basis with a variety of patients. Although increased attention is currently being directed to the psychosocial aspects of child health care, any substantial increase in these efforts will require additional funding, a highly unlikely development. In addition to deterrents within training programs, the problem also derives from a restricted perception by trainees and practitioners of their professional role. Such professional identity can be positively influenced by admired role models and by what is done in an educational setting (that is, human aggregate factors). However, it seems to me that the trainees must assume much of the responsibility to develop *on their own* the capacity to integrate and deliver simultaneously both those affective and the technical aspects of care that are essential for adequate communication. Whereas such self-responsibility for communication cannot reasonably be expected from all patients, it is a personal obligation of all health professionals. Lack of time and inadequate reimbursement are, of course, deterrents, but better communication can be accomplished in the time now available.

It is important that each of us in our own way and in our own setting persist in a wide variety of efforts to make more visible what needs to be accomplished and to demonstrate through teaching, patient care, and research how communication in child health services can be enhanced. This Pediatric Round Table is dedicated to that goal.

Morris Green, M.D.
Perry W. Lesh Professor and Chairman
Department of Pediatrics
Indiana University School of Medicine
Indianapolis, Indiana

INTRODUCTION

As we rapidly approach the 21st century, it may be well to take stock of where we as a nation have come from and where we are going in the delivery of health care services. When one looks at health care systems in this country, one immediately becomes aware of a perception by some of growing dissatisfaction among the lay public. While some of this dissatisfaction may be attributed to rising health care costs, another major reason appears to be inadequate communication between health professionals and the people in their care. As a result of poor or faulty communication, many people (from 15 to an astounding 95 percent, as reported by Rosenberg), do not follow physicians' instructions, and many others have filed lawsuits against health professionals.

Effective communication between health professionals and patients is complicated, and when the patient is a child it is even more complicated. Communicating effectively about the care of children is particularly challenging because of the need to involve both children and parents, because of the varying levels of understanding that children have at different ages, and because of the change in the kinds of health problems with which children are presenting. Once, health professionals who cared for children spent most of their time treating acute illnesses. However, today children present with an increasing number of psychosocial problems, chronic and fatal illnesses, and handicapping conditions — all of which require more professional time for counseling and for sensitive and insightful listening and communicating.

The reasons for ineffective communication between health professionals and children and their parents are many. One major reason is that the public sees the role of the health provider as not only diagnosing disease but also relieving suffering. (Suffering, as used here, refers not only to physical pain, but also to mental anguish.) Yet medical schools have traditionally concentrated on the former, in part because it is seen as more concrete and therefore easier to evaluate. Medical schools tend to select bright students who have demonstrated that they can acquire knowledge, but the schools give scant attention to students' potential for learning effective interpersonal communication skills. In addition, throughout medical education, the biological nature of living organisms is being increasingly dissected into its smallest elements. In fact, recent advances in cellular and molecular biology exceed what anyone might have imagined a few decades ago. As a result, students of medicine are required to learn an ever-increasing number of facts, many of which will never be employed in medical practice.

A task force of the Association of American Medical Colleges (AAMC), which currently is reviewing medical education in this country, has found that most of the nation's 67,000 medical students spend 30 to 40 hours per week in classrooms and laboratories, plus study time, so that they work 18 hours each day on the average. The result is that the students do not have time to develop as well-rounded human beings. Dr. Steven Muller, President of Johns Hopkins University who heads the AAMC's task force, is concerned that the system may not only be creating an undue fascination with technology, but may be dehumanizing the students.

In addition to communication problems which result from the way physicians are trained, are problems which result from the way that health services are organized and paid for in this country. In almost all instances, there is a lack of third-party reimbursement for time spent in communication. Financial rewards — instead of being awarded to those who communicate effectively and thus alleviate human suffering — are given to those who perform the most medical procedures.

This Pediatric Round Table came about because those of us asked to be its architects believed that major improvements in the health status of children cannot be brought about without effective communication. Furthermore, we were of the opinion that child health care communication could and must be improved. Finally, we believed that effective communication to promote child health requires that everyone play a role; this includes the parents, children, physicians, nurses, and the entire range of community health and human service providers.

Working from these assumptions, we organized the Round Table to consider a number of issues. These included: the need for effective communication; methods of meeting specific needs; and broadly based strategies to approach the identified problems. Before concluding the brief three-day Round Table, persons attending (which included nurses, physicians, parents, advocates, and policy-makers) were requested to draft guidelines for effective communications. Their efforts are contained in Appendix A.

Prior to the Round Table, an effort was undertaken to develop descriptions of programs and projects which have addressed themselves to one or more aspects of effective communication to enhance child health. The communications examples which resulted were originally intended for use by Round Table participants only, but because it was hoped that they might be of interest to others, they have been published separately. Appendix B contains samples of these communications examples.

A number of people were especially helpful in preparation of this publication. Lisbeth Bamberger Schorr's insightful presentation concisely summarized the highlights of the Round Table; in addition, she gave thoughtful attention to the content and wording of the communication guidelines and the communications examples. Others who reviewed the guidelines and examples in detail include Ellen Perrin, Evan Charney, Robert Pantell, Mary Ann Lewis, and Robert Chamberlin. We are grateful for their time and assistance. Finally, our thanks to Jolene Constance, who patiently typed and re-typed the manuscript for this publication.

The editors realize that the efforts of this Round Table have been limited, and that some persons who have spent many years working in this field could not attend. It is our anticipation that this edition will be neither the definitive word nor the final conclusion as to how effective communication may be brought about. Instead, this publication represents our concern and the concern of others that much more needs to be done to promote effective health care communication and to thus improve the overall health and development of this nation's children.

William K. Frankenburg, M.D.
Director, Rocky Mountain
Child Development Center
University of Colorado
School of Medicine
Denver, Colorado

PART I
AREAS OF NEED FOR IMPROVED HEALTH CARE COMMUNICATION

The papers included in Part I address a wide range of issues involving communication which impacts child health. As soon becomes apparent to anyone who delves into this area, "communication" as a topic is difficult to address because it involves so many variables, including interactions of children with parents, children and parents with health professionals, and health professionals with other health professionals. The presentations touch on all these interactions and go further to outline the special communication and service needs of children who are poor, chronically ill, or handicapped. In addition, the authors address problems within the health care system which have a negative impact on communication for child health.

Andrew Selig stresses the need for health professionals to understand and communicate with not only the child, but the child's entire family. He defines "family" as including parents, siblings, grandparents, and significant others. If the family is not actively involved in planning for the child's care, Selig emphasizes, health care plans and treatment recommendations may be inappropriate and are likely to be ignored.

Lorna Facteau believes that young children — even infants — have the potential for self-care, and that this potential should be encouraged. If children's self-monitoring behaviors are developed, she says, they will be more likely to take responsibility for their own health as they grow older. Facteau touches on what was to become a recurring controversy during the Round Table: How much responsibility should be assigned for communication regarding health care to children and parents, and how much responsibility should rest with health professionals?

Since 1940, Barbara Korsch's research has focused on communication between health professionals and patients. She describes highlights of her work and concludes that effective communication is not intuitive. Instead, she believes that communication processes can be researched and that communication skills can be taught.

Ellen Perrin's fascinating presentation describes how children understand the workings of their bodies and how they understand illness. Perrin notes that children's understanding develops in stages and over time. She says it is essential for health professionals to know the child's level of understanding if effective communication is to occur.

Robert Pantell echoes Perrin's conviction that professionals must understand children's levels of understanding to communicate effectively. He presents the benefits of preparing children for hospitalization and painful medical procedures, and describes some innovative preparation approaches.

The needs of chronically ill children and their families are addressed by Michael Weitzman. His paper focuses on the special needs of chronically ill children, and notes that too often medical specialization results in fragmentation of services. He states the need for long-term continuity of care and for coordination of services for these children. When he wrote of his belief that the coordinator of services should be a pediatrician, Weitzman raised issues which reoccurred throughout the Round Table: Is coordination and communication with the family best provided by a pediatrician, or by some other professional or professionals? And should the role of the pediatrician be as a generalist or specialist?

Another group of children with special needs are children with handicapping conditions. Suzie Rimstidt and Kelley MacDonald, both who have had children with disabilities, present parents' perspectives. Rimstidt describes her experiences and those of other parents with health professionals in moving terms, and makes recommendations to professionals for both communication and caring. MacDonald discusses the substantial contributions which groups of parents can make when they work together. She describes one innovative parents' group which has brought about changes in legislation, improvements in insurance coverage and services in schools, and so on.

Jean Elder, Commissioner of the Agency for Developmental Disabilities, describes the evolution of the federal definition of "developmental disabilities," notes that this definition is used to determine who receives services, and discusses the difficulties of applying the definition to very young children. She describes the role of her agency in planning and in mobilizing and coordinating resources for the developmentally disabled.

Systems which serve the developmentally disabled are the focus of Jon Ziarnik's presentation. He points out that physicians are no longer the major care providers for handicapped persons. Instead, with the developmentally disabled moving out of institutions and into the community, teams of health and human service workers plan and provide services for individuals with handicaps.

Robert Chamberlin also discusses problems within systems — in this case, the systems which deliver health care to children. He states that poor children often don't receive the preventive or treatment services they need. Public health services are often so fragmented, he says, that it is impossible to provide care to meet all a child's needs. In addition, health services to poor children are of low priority in our society and so are usually eliminated first during times of budget cutbacks. Chamberlin emphasizes the need for community-based planning and coordination for health services.

Susan M. Thornton, M.S.

THE NEED FOR A FAMILY ORIENTATION

Andrew L. Selig, M.S.W., Sc.D.
and Ellen W. Selig, M.Ed.

All families have certain needs which a health care provider should strive to fulfill in order to provide quality health care. This is especially true when the patient is a child. These needs could be met if the health professional would do the following things. First, the professional should see the child in the context of the whole family unit and should try to understand the various influences on that child. Second, the professional should strive to understand a family's dynamics and patterns of interactions. Third, the professional should attempt to involve the family as much as possible in planning and in carrying out the child's treatment. And fourth, the professional should attempt to understand the family's basic value systems which are relevant to health care. The degree to which these needs can be fulfilled will vary, of course, according to the caregiver's specialty and/or role in the patient's life. The primary caregiver (for example, a family practitioner, pediatrician, public health nurse, etc.) should view these needs as of primary importance, while another specialist (such as an orthopedist or dermatologist) would probably not become as involved with the needs, depending on the situation.

The Effects of Fragmentation and Poor Communication on the Family and Its Members

The development of health specialties and subspecialties is the result of increasing medical knowledge, improvements, and sophistication. In general, we all have benefited from this increasing specialization and knowledge. However, two basic problem areas have emerged as a result of these new trends: fragmentation of care and poor communication.

Specialists, by the very nature of their training and work, are concerned with smaller and smaller aspects of functioning, often ignoring other aspects of the child, who needs to be seen not only as a total person but also as a member of a total family. When the caregiver treats only one small part of the patient (for example, a stomach ache or an allergy) and does not make an effort to become aware of what else is going on with the child and family, the problem may be misdiagnosed and/or incorrectly treated. Health professionals must become aware that a thorough understanding of the family and their dynamics is basic to understanding the child and planning interventions, as well as to the success of those interventions.

Problems in communication stemming from specialization of the health care system can be viewed in several ways. The family may not know to which caregiver they should turn for a given problem, the caregiver may not speak to the real problem, or the caregiver may not speak in a way that can be understood by the child or family. When a number of caregivers are involved with a given family — as is often the case — communication is often misdirected or haphazard; even worse, faulty information is often given or received. One caregiver may not be aware of another's involvement, or may not know that other problems exist, and may therefore treat a problem in a vacuum. Specialists may also not feel they have the time — or even the need — to try to understand a family's dynamics or communication patterns, and may therefore not communicate with them in a way that can be understood or be relevant. Thus, a specialist may miss the real causes of a problem, may not understand that a child's "problem" is actually a symptom of a larger family problem, or may not realize that a course of treatment for an individual child is actually becoming a problem for the family as a whole.

Of course, not only specialists may be guilty of fragmentation and miscommunication. Primary health providers may also find communication difficult. A case was recently referred to me that helps illustrate these points.

> The family consists of a mother, father, and two sons (ages 12 and 8). The mother had just returned from a visit to her pediatrician where she had been told that her son needed individual psychotherapy. She was very upset about this recommendation and questioned the physician's judgment. The physician, as part of a routine annual examination, asked the child questions about his relationships with friends and members of the family. The child stated, in a rather shy and reticent manner, that he did not get along very well with his father. At this point, the physician was called out of the room by a nurse who asked him to look at another child. When the pediatrician came back

into the room he did not continue with his questioning but, instead, recommended psychotherapy for the child. The mother felt that the physician had not accurately assessed the situation and had failed to gather information on the family and the child's substantial strengths. The mother felt strongly that the physician understood only part of what was going on with her son.

The Importance of Family Dynamics in Understanding the Child

To understand the influence of the family on the child's health and development, professionals need to study the family's dynamics from the point of view of parental, marital, sibling, and extended family relationships. There are many parenting styles, which all affect a child's personality development in one way or another. For example, a parent can be overly permissive, overly protective, too disinterested, or too domineering; each of these tendencies would be reflected in a child's physical, emotional, and behavioral development.

The quality of the marital system has been shown to be directly related to the quality of parenting. When continual and unresolved tension persists in the marriage, there is a higher than average probability that the parents will focus attention on a child (or children) to relieve the stress in their marriage. For example, marital tension can lead parents to continually see "problems" in a particular child, and can lead to them devoting substantial amounts of time and energy to helping that child. This serves to divert attention from their troubled marriage.

Understanding the sibling system within the family also helps the professional understand any particular child. In the example just mentioned, a sibling may become very resentful of the child who receives undue attention, and may act out or develop symptoms as a way to get attention from the parents. It has been shown that sibling position and sex alone have profound effects on personality development. For example, middle children often have a more difficult time finding a way to receive recognition and attention within their family than oldest or youngest children. In some family contexts, the oldest child is expected to — and often does — take parental responsibility for younger siblings; in such a case, the position within the family system can lead to the "parentified" child never really experiencing childhood.

Relationships with extended family members are also very important in understanding family dynamics. Some of the more powerful influences on any family are the past and current experiences and relationships that the parents had and have with their own families of origin. Grandparents can exert tremendous influence over all aspects of their children's and grandchildren's lives. For example, it is not unusual for a grandparent to recognize a child's difficulties within the family, and for the grandparent to make a special effort to help that child. This can sometimes be beneficial, but in some cases it can cause problems.

Another possible problem area is the parents' inadequate emotional separation from their families of origin. This can lead to so much over-involvement by grandparents in their children's families that the development of a strong commitment between spouses is continually undermined. Understanding the complex relationships with extended family members can often be the key to understanding behavior and attitudes within a nuclear family.

These four basic areas of family dynamics — the quality of the parental relationship, of the marital relationship, of the sibling relationships, and of the relationships with extended family — can all influence the health of individual family members. Health professionals should always be aware that a child can develop a symptom which is actually only a "cry for help," a cry that something else has actually gone awry in the family system.

The family dynamics in the family mentioned previously can help illustrate by a case example some of the points made.

> The mother agrees that her younger son (for whom psychotherapy was recommended) has difficulties, and that his self-concept is low. The father, who is very athletic and derives a lot of pride and self-confidence from his own athletic endeavors, is very negative and critical of the younger son who is not very athletic. Their older son is good at sports, which tends to promote more closeness between the father and older son, and to distance the younger child that much more. Other dynamics that help explain the behavior in the identified patient are also at work in this family. The mother and father argue constantly about parenting their children. The father complains that the mother is much too lenient with the younger child, and that she constantly makes excuses for his behavior (including his hesitancy in athletic endeavors). The mother, on the other hand, is very critical of her husband for being so critical toward their younger son. Each feels the other is being a "bad parent," and each tries

to compensate for what they feel the other is lacking in their respective relationships with their sons.

Understanding the dynamics in this family in their entirety would increase communication and make the possibility of a successful intervention more likely. Ideally, each family member would work on his or her own part of the process; this would tremendously increase the probability for significant and rapid changes to benefit the identified child.

The Importance of Family Dynamics in Planning and Carrying Out Treatment

An understanding of a family's dynamics is also important in planning treatment interventions. An extremely well-conceived treatment plan for a child can meet with failure if the process of the evaluation and treatment planning does not "mesh" with the needs and values of a child's family. That is one reason it is important to include a family assessment as part of most diagnostic procedures for a child, since it helps understand the context in which the family (and therefore the child) lives. In addition, a family assessment tells the family that the health provider is interested in and values their perceptions. Such an assessment communicates in both subtle and overt ways the professional's recognition of the importance that other family members play in the child's life. When family members are part of the process that arrives at findings, there is increased likelihood that they will feel identified with those findings, and that they will pursue interventions.

The case example of the family in my practice can help illustrate the importance of involving the family in diagnosis and treatment planning.

> The family has seen numerous physicians over the last several years and "shopped" from physician to physician because of their dissatisfaction with each one. Both the mother and father are overweight, and the father smokes a great deal. All the physicians to whom they have gone — including family physicians from whom they have sought services for the whole family — have told the parents that they need to lose weight and that the father needs to stop smoking. The father has responded to this advice angrily, and when the physicians have continued to push for change, the father has decided time after time that he was

not going to return.

In my first consultation with the family, it became clear that any future health provider would once again lose the family if he or she did not understand their reluctance to change. The family's felt need, which at the time I first saw them was dealing with the pediatrician's recommendation for psychotherapy for their younger son, is of primary importance. It is the one need to which initial attention should be directed. At times, even though the provider sees the importance of other needs, he or she must sometimes "let ride" issues with which the family is not yet ready to deal.

The Importance of the Family's Basic Value Systems as They Relate to Child Health Care

All families have basic values and attitudes toward health and illness, and toward seeking medical care. The more the health care provider understands these value orientations, the greater the probability that the care provider will communicate appropriately and responsively to the family's needs.

There are several very important areas where value orientations play a role in health care. One is the question of where the responsibility for the health of family members lies. Some parents do not feel that prevention, healthy lifestyles, and good health habits are necessary. They usually put the health care provider in the role of "God," and when something is wrong with one of the family members they "get treated," but continue their irresponsible lifestyle. This attitude places the entire responsibility for maintaining health on the shoulders of the health professional.

Another closely aligned attitude is the degree to which a parent or family member wishes to be involved in treatment planning, or even to be informed of what the situation is. Some people feel that the health care provider — as "God" — knows all, and they will do whatever the professional feels is necessary. Others ask many questions, demand to be involved, and are mistrustful of a health care provider who does not support their involvement.

Other important values are those of the family's attitude toward dependency and toward assuming the patient role. Some feel that it is undesirable to be in this role, and put pressure on a child to "carry on" and not complain; others give so much attention to physical ailments that they almost encourage a child to become a hypochondriac.

Another related attitude involves feelings about medication. Some families feel that medicine should be administered only if seen as really necessary or only if a person is in extreme pain; the extreme of this would be avoiding giving a child medication even when it is definitely needed. Others feel better just knowing that medication is being given, even if it is not totally necessary. They also might take painkillers at the slightest symptom, and may feel that people should be spared from suffering any discomfort at all. These people may not consider possible drug side effects, or may not understand the danger of some drug interactions.

The health professional who does not understand a family's values in these four areas would find it very difficult to effectively treat a child within the context of the family. The treatment might not fit the family's framework and would therefore be something that the family could not follow. (In some cases, if it becomes apparent that the family's and professional's values are too dissimilar, the health provider may even need to refer the family to someone else.)

The case example previously mentioned illustrates the importance of the health care provider's understanding of a family's values.

> The family demands a great deal of involvement with the health care provider in both making the diagnosis and in suggesting treatment. The mother was very hesitant to follow through on the physician's recommendation for individual psychotherapy since she did not believe that the physician adequately understood the issues (and had not asked her opinion).

This family is not likely to take the advice of a care provider without feeling that their needs and thoughts have been carefully heard and considered. Although this mother and father both are well aware of the potential problems with their being overweight and smoking, their self-determination values lead them to resent health care providers who continue to push them to deal with these issues when they are not ready to do so themselves. Any future health care provider is more likely to successfully work with this family if he or she understands this kind of thinking and works *with* it, rather than directly confronting it.

In conclusion, families have certain needs that should be met in order to improve communication and to ensure high-quality health care for their children. In addition, it should be emphasized that the family — and especially the parents — have a responsibility to express their needs as much as health care providers have a responsibility to meet them. If family members sit back passively, without actively taking a role in communication, they are as much to blame for poor quality health care as the professional.

To try to meet the family's needs, health care providers should do the following. They should ask many questions, especially in a way that makes family members feel comfortable and encourages them to reveal information. They should be aware of other health and human service providers involved with the family, and should communicate with these other providers when necessary. They should see the child in the context of the whole family unit, and try to understand the various influences on the child. They should encourage family involvement in the child's diagnostic and treatment procedures. And finally, professionals should try to understand the family's values; when these are too dissimilar to their own, the professional should refer the family to another provider.

DISCUSSION

Jon Ziarnik: I am wondering at what point there is a trade-off between the professional's responsibility and the consumer's responsibility. For example, perhaps the mother you talked about should have said to the physician, "I am very unhappy with your recommendations for psychotherapy for my child."

Andy Selig: I think that raises an important point. Consumers certainly do have some responsibility. Your question makes me think that in a way I might have failed the mother. Maybe the best suggestion I could have given her would have been to go back and talk to the pediatrician with her complaint. Perhaps I became part of the problem rather than the solution by not doing that.

Lorna Facteau: But expecting consumers to be assertive is more easily said than done. You are expecting a lot of patients to expect them to be assertive.

Chuck Lewis: Consumers can be taught to be assertive, but we have found that it does take training.

Lee Schorr: For a moment I was afraid that Jon might be suggesting that the parent has the task of making up for what the physician was not taught in medical school or residency training. It seems to me that a mother can go through assertiveness training and say to the physician, "Look, I don't feel too good about what you just told me." But unless the physician has the capacity for sensitivity and communication, parental assertiveness is not going to be very effective.

Mary Ann Lewis: The point Andy made with which I agree is that physicians might be able to provide better services if they understood systems theory. They could not only be more efficient, but they would also be more effective in regard to prevention.

Andy Selig: What really has surprised me in my experience with physicians is that they do learn systems. For example, they learn that a systems approach is a major part of thinking about how the body functions. But when it comes to thinking about systems outside the workings of our bodies, they stop. Physicians just are not taught about systems in regard to interpersonal relationships.

Bob Pantell: It has been my experience that when I start asking probing questions about family interactions, role expectations come into play. These expectations come from patients' traditional interractions with physicians, I believe. For example, pediatricians usually just focus on the child. So when pediatricians start asking about interactions between the parents, some parents are not willing to respond. It seems to me that family practitioners almost have a license to ask some of these questions, that parents are more willing to have family physicians probe sensitive areas. The point is that more than training of professionals is involved. We've all got to prepare patients to accept a systems level of intervention.

Joy Penticuff: I would like to make a point about the transient nature of relationships within health care systems which I think is very important in understanding the situation that Andy described. The family who came to him was a family with a tendency to shop around, yet relationships in which people are willing to be forthcoming about what is going on in their family take time. I would wonder a little about the long-term effects of assertiveness training. I could see that ultimately it might have positive outcomes, but I think there has to be a relationship over time between the physician and the family if real sharing and understanding are to develop.

Evan Charney: Andy, I think my first reaction to your story was that the physician was an insensitive clod and that the mother should not pay her bill. But on reflection, I think what happened was more complex. It seems to me that the crucial test is whether or not the physician can respond when the parent comes back and challenges the recommendation for psychotherapy. It is possible that the physician made exactly the right recommendation given complex circumstances, but it is also possible that the physician did not make the right recommendation. Perhaps the physician was usually very sensitive and generally was capable of establishing good relationships. We do not know what happened in the next room; perhaps it was something upsetting, so that the physician was not as sensitive as usual. If this is true, the system just needs a little course correction by the mother challenging him. I think we won't know unless the mother is able to take the next step. If she runs and leaves the system, the problem may go on.

I am also troubled at how to develop families' abilities to challenge physicians, because if we do not develop assertiveness skills, we won't have good communication. While I am troubled about how to increase family skills, where it has been done, I have seen that mountains move and systems change. Without such change, I think you are dealing with only half of the equation.

THE NEED TO TEACH SELF-CARE SKILLS

Lorna M. Facteau, R.N., M.S.

Promoting health in childhood is a common goal among health care professionals, and teaching self-care skills to children is a means to this end. While children may vary in their self-care abilities depending on age, even a young child can engage in some self-care activities. In fact, clinical experience demonstrates that children will engage in some aspects of self-care depending not only on their age and developmental level, but also depending on cultural and familial influences.

In this paper, I will briefly present a framework for self-care, describe the potentials for self-care among infants and toddlers, and discuss parents' responsibilities. Finally, I will address the need for professionals to teach self-care to children as a way to prevent major chronic diseases.

Definition of Self-Care

Self-care is defined by Orem as the activities of individuals that are initiated and performed on their own behalf in maintaining life, health, and well-being. There are several assumptions on which this self-care concept is based:

- The human being is adaptive, creative, and integrated with the environment.
- Self-care behaviors are learned relative to beliefs, habits, and practices indigenous to the group to which the individual belongs.
- Self-care behaviors are positive, practical, and deliberate; in regard to health, self-care behaviors are goal-oriented toward wellness.

Orem describes two major categories of self-care. One type is considered universal, and includes basic human requirements for air, food, water, shelter, rest, and socialization. The other category includes behaviors required only in the event of an illness or developmental life-cycle event. A factor important to either category of self-care behaviors is motivation.

Within Orem's model, infants and children require care from others because they are in the early stages of development physically, psychologically, and psychosocially. Care for others is the adult's (parent's) contribution to the health and well-being of the dependent members (children) of their social group (family). The limitation of this model is that it negates infants' and toddlers' potential for self-care.

Potentials for Self-Care in Infants and Toddlers

Children's self-care abilities are based on a variety of factors. These include developmental and emotional levels, familial and cultural influences, and cognitive and motor skills. As a child learns and grows, the potential for self-care increases and new skills are learned and old ones are refined.

To the casual observer, the newborn seems totally helpless and dependent on others for protection, comfort, and nurturing. However, even the youngest infants have signaling behaviors in their repertoire of expression. These signaling actions stimulate the parent to act to fulfill the infant's needs.

The infant's potentials for self-care are based upon a complex set of perceptual and reflex capacities. Among other findings, research has shown that:

- the infant prefers the human face to other designs;

- the infant is programmed to move in rhythm to the human voice;
- the infant orients with his or her eyes, head, and body to animate sounds; and
- the infant alerts with human holding and rocking.

These capacities permit the infant to engage in interactive human relationships which form a basis for exploration and learning that are the foundation for self-care behaviors.

While the infant's abilities can be described in primitive terms, they are nonetheless significant to self-care. The infant signals (by crying) for food in response to an empty stomach. Thus, the action is deliberate and oriented toward maintaining life and well-being; yet, in infancy, the cognitive content of this behavior is limited.

Throughout the first year, development enables the infant to expand other self-care activities. The behaviors which result in self-feeding are an example. The infant begins with haphazard hand-arm movements. By four months, these movements are coordinated so that the infant can get the hands to midline and then bring them to the mouth. At six months, torso control enables the child to maintain a sitting position. As the first year progresses, the combination of these sophisticated behaviors facilitates self-feeding.

During the toddler years, the child's autonomy increases. Developmental milestones include language acquisition and toileting behaviors, among others.

The development of language is important to self-care, for language helps the child communicate with others directly. As the toddler's nonverbal "signals" are turned into words, the child is able to ask directly for assistance with self-care.

The behaviors which facilitate toileting are as complex as those which lead to the development of language. The refinement of gross and fine motor control along with sphincter control, language development, and emotional readiness enable the child to accomplish the self-care task of toileting.

As the development of language and toileting demonstrates, the process that prepares a child for independence and increases activities toward self-care starts at birth and continues through childhood. At every stage of development, children show their specific potentials and abilities for self-care. These behaviors of self-care are more than the simple execution of motor skills. Rather, they are a set of sophisticated behaviors that include physical, perceptual motor, and cognitive skills as well as constitutional drives and self-concept.

Parental Considerations

Children require varying degrees of help with self-care activities depending on their developmental level. Parents, who provide this help, find that the nature of the assistance changes quantitatively, as well as qualitatively, as the child grows.

In infancy, parents provide for children's basic needs. The parent who wishes to foster self-care lets the infant regulate him- or herself by responding to signals from the infant rather than presuming the infant's need. In this way, the parent begins to teach the child healthy life-style patterns of self-care behavior. During the toddler years, parents continue to foster self-care behavior in their children by encouraging the child's autonomy and independence.

The Need to Teach Self-Care

The need to teach children self-care is based on the frequent finding that unhealthy life-style habits are established in childhood. These habits (precursory self-care behaviors) are mediated by parents within the context of the family's sociocultural beliefs. Because childhood is the time when unhealthy patterns are often established, it is an appropriate time to implement primary prevention programs to decrease risk for chronic diseases.

During infancy and the toddler years, behavior is the essence of teaching aspects of self-care. The young child's cognitive level prevents the use of programs aimed at increasing the level of knowledge, although cognitive content must be included for parents at this time. Social learning and behavioral models are more suited for children in this age group.

One example of how teaching self-care during early childhood could decrease the incidence of a health problem involves obesity. Research has found that overweight infants tend to become overweight children and adolescents, who in turn become overweight adults. Most experts agree that obesity is the result of a combination of problems, including metabolic abnormalities, poor understanding of nutrition, limited physical activity, and inappropriate response to stress (among others). Thus, self-care teaching protocols for parents of infants and toddlers might include topics such as nutritional requirements in early childhood, extra-nutritional sucking needs of infants, behavioral capabilities in infancy, and so on.

In summary, children at every developmental level exhibit both potentials and abilities for self-care. Since these self-care behaviors — life-style habits — tend to be enduring, primary prevention programs involving self-care teaching protocols for children and their parents are appropriate and can help reduce future health risks.

DISCUSSION

Mary Ann Lewis: I would challenge the concept of self-care as you define it because it does not stress self-motivation and decision-making. To my mind, self-care denotes that one takes deliberate action rather than being a self-regulatory mechanism that occurs because of physiologic response to the environment.

Lee Schorr: Why do you put the two-way communication between parent and infant in the category of self-care? Why don't you put your emphasis on helping parents respond to infants?

Lorna Facteau: I do this basically because I believe that infants have a very strong part in forming their environments. If we focus on parental responsibilities, we tend to have the sort of system that we have now, where infants are not seen as major contributors to their particular environment in terms of needs being met.

Chuck Lewis: I think there is some agreement among professionals that self-care could reduce health costs and improve health. But my experience is that most adults are not really interested in self-care. For example, Mary Ann and I just did a decision-making health curriculum which involves self-care for bumps and bruises in schools. We introduced it in 20 national classrooms, and found that the teachers did not like the self-care portion of the curriculum. And physicians are often terrible examples, perhaps because they do not want to give up control.

Jon Ziarnik: I would like to add that I see many community-based programs for the developmentally disabled which teach dependency. Teaching self-care would take away professionals' control. I think control is a big issue.

Earl Schaefer: I found in looking at parents' behavior with infants at four months and at one year, that the parents' initiatives, interactions, and stimulation predicted the child's academic competence in kindergarten years later. So I think we can overdo just emphasizing response to a child. The parent is active; the child is active. There is a dialogue going on.

Lorna Facteau: I would say that we are talking about a complementary relationship between parent and infant. The parent receives a signal, the infant gives a signal, and there is a complementary relationship.

Joy Penticuff: Lorna, it sounds to me like what you are saying is that what we need to do is not violate the self-regulating mechanisms of children, starting early, and that when we do violate those mechanisms, we are in trouble. In addition, I would like to state my belief that consumers need to have control within health care systems. For example, in Austin, Texas, there is a group of university-educated women who have decided to have their children at home; they are even deciding to be delivered by lay midwives instead of physicians. I think, from talking with these people, that their basic feeling is that they lose control in the health care system over what they see as a healthy process. We really must take to heart what you are talking about in terms of control. I feel that we must interact with consumers in such a way as to let the consumers know that they do have control.

Bob Pantell: I just want to make one comment: children are really vulnerable in this whole self-care issue. If we do an effective job of teaching children self-care skills, parents still make the decisions about when to seek medical care. It has been documented over and over again that families are far more likely to bring their children in when they are under periods of family stress, rather than when the child feels it is appropriate to see a physician.

Lorna Facteau: That is a good point. Clearly, we need to teach all members of the family.

DOCTOR-PATIENT COMMUNICATION IN ACUTE CHILD HEALTH CARE

Barbara M. Korsch, M.D.

For many years, communication between physicians and patients was considered part of the "art of medicine" and was thus believed to be an unsuitable subject for scientific inquiry. Students and trainees were expected to learn about communication skills from their senior colleagues by observation while they served an apprentice role. Most physicians have tended to pride themselves on their communication skills (their "bedside manner") and tend to feel very confident about their rapport with their patients. This confidence and pleasure in interaction are reinforced by the experience of many practitioners who care for patients who seek them out; over time these physicians tend to select a patient population with which they seem to feel comfortable communicating.

Unfortunately, the consumers of medical care have not been as pleased with the physicians' communication skills as physicians have liked to think. In recent years, there has been more dissatisfaction with the doctor-patient relationship and with physician-patient communication than with physicians' technical skills. Most frequently heard complaints in respect to medical care have been, "The doctor didn't understand," "The doctor didn't listen to me," "The doctor wasn't sensitive," and, "The doctor wasn't concerned." This kind of complaint is heard much more frequently than statements of discontent with the doctor's technical or diagnostic skills, or scientific knowledge. One cogent example of the degree of dissatisfaction with communication between physicians and their patients, as well as with doctor-patient relationships, can be found in an examination of malpractice suits. Many of these lawsuits are actually found to relate to poor physician communication rather than failure to practice appropriate technical medical skills.

Starting in the late 1940s and proceeding with increasing refinement and scope through the 1960s and '70s, our own research group responded to the challenge of learning about doctor-patient communications in a more scientific way. It was our conviction that the process of communication between physicians and their patients could be subject to scientific scrutiny; that it should be possible to analyze elements which make for either effective or ineffective communication; and that accumulating a body of scientific knowledge about this important area of medical care could be the basis for improved education, training, and practice. I would next like to briefly discuss a summary of some of the research data we have obtained over time.

A Major Doctor-Patient Communication Study

After various smaller and less ambitious projects to study breakdowns in doctor-patient communications, our group received a very large research grant in the mid-'60s from the (then) Children's Bureau in Washington. We established a study with a sufficiently large sample of doctor-patient encounters so that reliable and valid inferences concerning the communication process could be drawn. In designing this study, we attempted to select patient visits which would let us scrutinize the process of communication as undistorted as possible by extraneous factors. In order to achieve this goal, we decided to utilize first visits between patients and physicians; this helped eliminate the influence of previously existing relationships. We decided to study the first visit relating to a particular illness so that the patient's previous encounters around the illness would not distort the communication being studied, and we decided to include a wide variety of patient conditions so that the communication process could be studied in a general way, and not just as it related to a particular kind of complaint.

Approximately 1,000 visits were examined in this study, 800 of which were included in the definitive sample after some preliminary explorations. A subsequent validation study added another smaller number of patient visits for examination. Finally, in subsequent years, refinements (including videotapes) were added and smaller additional samples were studied in private practice settings.

The research methodology in the main project was essentially as follows. By random assignment, patients visiting an acute care walk-in clinic at Children's Hospital of Los Angeles were included in the sample. Informed consent was obtained from both the patient and health professional involved, and the entire medical encounter was recorded on audiotape. (An audiotape recorder was placed in each physician's office prior to the visit.) An interview was carried out immediately after the visit by a research associate with the child's mother, and within two weeks a follow-up interview was carried out by the same person. Our hypothesis was that there are attributes of the doctor-patient communication which influence the outcome of this communication. We measured this outcome originally in terms of three outcome variables: patient satisfaction, follow-through on medical advice (that is, compliance), and patient reassurance. Since it was found after analysis was begun that reassurance and satisfaction were highly correlated, the final results were reported in terms of patient satisfaction and compliance.

The interaction process was analyzed by a great many methods, some of which were developed as we went along, and some of which were adapted from other existing studies and situations. Among other features of the communication process, analysis was planned to include content of the interaction, sequence of the interaction, affect from both patient and physician during the interaction, and some formalistic components of the interaction process. One of the major approaches used was an adaptation of the Bales Interaction

Process Analysis, a method originally developed to study small group interactions.

Details of our various research projects have been published in a number of scientific journals, and I will not attempt to give you details here. However, since this is a meeting devoted to the communication between health professionals and their patients, I would like to briefly summarize some relevant findings. Our most important finding was that there was a strong correlation between the communication process and outcome in terms of satisfaction and compliance. Another, more surprising, finding was that the communication process was a stronger predictor of outcome than some of the features which had previously been thought to be of more fundamental importance (that is, the patient's demographic background, the nature of the illness around which the communication took place, and other elements of the situation or attributes of the patient and physician).

I must stress at this point that the situation which we studied in our research was a single encounter around an acute illness or a new problem, and that our follow-up was short-term. The literature suggests that there are a number of very cogent determinants of the effectiveness and use of health care, of the satisfaction with health care, and of people's health behavior which would become much more important when one looks at chronic illness and long-term doctor-patient relationships. The literature on health behavior, on compliance with medical advice, and on use of various health services is full of interesting and valid information on the social, cultural, psychological, and personality variables which influence the effectiveness of health care and the way in which it is delivered and accepted. There are interesting speculations and studies relating patient reactions to certain physician attributes. The barriers to health care, including financial barriers, also have been shown to make a difference to what goes on between patients and health care providers. However, for the purposes of this discussion, I will focus on the communication process as such — and specifically the communication process as it has been documented by our group — in respect to ambulatory health care of children with an acute illness.

Findings Regarding the Patient's Main Concern

Two main themes that kept emerging in every aspect of the study were: (1) the basic importance of eliciting and responding to patients' main concerns, not just the stated chief complaint, but also the underlying concern; and (2) the need to respond specifically to the patient's expectations for the encounter.

We were astonished to find that in more than 300 of 800 clinical encounters, the patient's main concern was never expressed in the course of the interaction, and that an even larger number of patients perceived that their main concerns had never been elicited, understood, or acknowledged by the physician. (Parenthetically, I must state that of course in studying pediatric practice, very often it is the patient's mother, or a responsible caretaker of the patient, whose concerns are the subject of discussion. In our substantive sample, we made a point of including no children above 10 years of age, because it would have complicated the research design to have to deal with the child's concerns as well as the concerns of the parent. Thus, when I refer to the "patient's concerns," it should be understood that the phrase is shorthand for alluding to the concerns of the mother or the caretaker.)

It was very easy to elicit these underlying concerns during the post-visit interview by having a public health nurse or research assistant ask a few simple questions (for example, "Why did you bring your child to the doctor today? What worried you the most about that? Why did that worry you?"). Such questions might reveal that the child had been brought in with a fever, that what worried the mother most was that the fever was so high, and that she wondered why it didn't decrease with aspirin. Finally, when asked why the continuation of the fever worried her, the mother might respond that she had heard that children sometimes get convulsions from high fevers. If this concern had not been discussed during the interaction with the physician, the mother would tend to feel poorly understood, would be less satisfied with her visit, and would be less prone to follow the physician's advice.

Eliciting the patient's expectations from the visit was also a simple process. It was more difficult to deal with these expectations, since patient's expectations are often unrealistic. Some parents want their child hospitalized when this is not medically required, and some want antibiotic prescriptions or penicillin injections for virus infections. Thus, it is not always possible to deal with the patient's expectations simply by satisfying them. It was our experience, however, that if the expectation had been elicited, and if the physician was able to meaningfully bridge what the patient's expectation had been and what the physician was or was not doing, the patient would be satisfied.

Other Findings

Another attribute of the communication process which our study showed to be a significant predictor of patient satisfaction and follow-through was the amount of positive affect expressed by the physician toward the parent. Thus, it was discouraging to find that a relatively low percentage of physicians' interactions with mothers demonstrated positive effect. In some portions of the study, only five percent of the physician's communication to the mother could be classified as being friendly, although more than 40 percent of the communication between the child and doctor tended to be friendly. This is probably a reflection of the pediatrician's tendency to identify strongly with the child and to not feel as closely allied with the child's mother as might be desirable.

One surprising finding was that the time of the interaction was not specifically correlated with the outcome. We found that very short interactions could lead to satisfaction and compliance, while long ones — in some instances — were actually suggestive of poor communication. Interactions in which the mother failed to enlist the doctor's interest in her concerns tended to be long; visits were prolonged as physician and patient each talked on their own wave length instead of finding a common ground for communication. Another finding which to our surprise was statistically significant was that the presence of even a small amount of non-medical, non-task-oriented communication between physician and patient was statistically correlated with patient satisfaction. It seemed that when a child's mother was acknowledged as a person in her own right and offered the courtesy of some response to herself as a person (not simply as the caretaker of a sick child), she responded with increased satisfaction and cooperation.

In the first sample of recorded doctor-patient interactions, the overall incidence of high satisfaction was 40 percent, and compliance was 42 percent. There was no significant difference in compliance with different kinds of medication. There was a high correlation between satisfaction and cooperation with medical advice, but of interest to us was that there were a number of patients who were highly dissatisfied who *did* follow through on all the advice offered, and there were some highly satisfied patients who did *not* follow through with the doctor's recommendations. There was a tendency for patients and families who felt that they had been given an inadequate explanation of diagnosis or etiology to be highly dissatisfied. There was a general tendency for the physicians to participate more actively in interactions than mothers; this was true even though many of the physicians felt that they had allowed the mothers full expression, and many felt they had done far more listening than talking.

There were interesting instances in which communication seemed to break down totally. What we found was a particular point in the interaction, which came when the mother had made various attempts to engage the physician on behalf of her concerns or perceptions of the illness, when the mother finally gave up. Subsequently, mothers indicated that after they had given up hope of achieving true communication, they no longer heard what the physician had said or even perceived physical manipulations of the child.

In general, the study showed that mothers were good reporters of what had indeed gone on between them and the physicians, and that our objective analyses of the interaction content and process were fairly well mirrored in the mothers' perceptions. Obviously, there were exceptions to this generalization.

This study design was not suitable to analyze differences in individual doctor's styles or effectiveness. A large number of physicians were involved, and there were not a sufficient number of cases per doctor for each one to display a particular communication style or effectiveness. To the extent that the analyses were carried out, we found that every physician in the sample was more effective with certain kinds of problems than with others, and that no one was able to achieve effective communication across the board. It was also interesting to find that, within the limited sample of doctors, increased experience did not result in improved communication techniques. However, in general, we found that the private practice setting did apparently lead to more ideal circumstances for communication and for mutual selection on the part of the physician and patient. As a result, although the same communication breakdowns were observed in private practice as in an institutional setting, the frequency of dissatisfaction was not as high in private practice.

The question as to whether other health professionals are more effective in their communication than physicians is often raised. Our studies do not contain the answer to this question; however, we did do a limited study with pediatric nurse practitioners conducting well baby care in which we observed the same phenomena and some of the same limitations as we did in the physician encounters.

The message that we carried away from these studies and have tried to share with interested health care workers is that the communication process is of tremendous importance in health care delivery. Even in short-term relationships relating to a particular acute illness, health behavior will be markedly affected by the way in which the physician approaches the patient. We found that the findings and case illustrations collected were easily adapted for teaching purposes, and they have been generally well accepted by trainees in various settings.

Examples of Physician-Patient Communications

Clinical encounters that our group has videotaped illustrate some of the significant attributes of doctor-patient communication uncovered in our study. The first case is that of a mother of a child with hypoglycemia who shows that her trust in the physician and consultants in the entire medical establishment is absolute; she feels that her physicians know what they are doing, and she believes all that they tell her. This mother demonstrates that in certain instances the patient comes nine-tenths of the way toward establishing a good relationship, and that there are patients who are ready to communicate and operate in a positive way.

The next example is a very poignant vignette dealing with an older black man who suffers from chronic emphysema and bronchitis, and who has just recovered from a lung abscess. He is talking to a young, white, female physician in a clinic setting. At the end of the physical examination, the young woman inquires briefly about the man's eating habits, and learns that he has a rather poor appetite and does not eat regularly. She then proceeds swiftly and briskly to ask him to make her two promises: (1) to eat three meals a day; and (2) to quit smoking. She makes these requests as the patient is tucking his shirt into his trousers; he is standing, and she is sitting at a desk writing in his chart. This vignette dramatically demonstrates some problems in eliciting patient cooperation: there was a large social distance between the patient and physician, and there was a poor clinical setting in that the patient was uncomfortable and preoccupied, while the physician was tending to her institutional business. In addition, asking a patient to change lifelong habits after only a brief encounter and without sufficient awareness of obstacles to compliance is unlikely to be productive. In this instance, the result of the interaction is clearly evident because the patient fails to promise to either eat three meals a day or to stop smoking. He simply says that he will do the best he can with the food, but that he will *not* stop smoking.

The third videotaped illustration deals with a physician who demonstrates a remarkable degree of tolerance for a patient's ideas concerning her own health care. It is a situation in which a young South American woman, who has been given a limited number of prescriptions for anticoagulants and hypertension as well as cardiac medication, arrives at the clinic with a sack full of variegated medicaments. She has brought these from healers in other cultures. The physician accepts this unexpected therapeutic regimen with a great deal of tolerance, and does not scold the woman or make her feel embarrassed for her self-medication.

The fourth example on videotape demonstrates a series of monotonous inquiries from a physician to a cardiac patient which can be answered only yes or no. This approach obviously leads to no communication whatsoever, and makes it impossible for the patient to express anything that is of significance to him. Throughout the interview, the physician looks at the chart, does not call the patient by name, and pays not a moment of attention to the patient as a person.

The fifth example documents a frequently observed phenomenon — namely, that physicians become uncomfortable when patients express emotions, and will escape from these by launching into neutral technological discussion. In this instance, the patient expresses how excited and upset she is about her daughter, and the physician interrupts by asking about her diuretic medication.

Two additional examples deal with adolescent patients. The first is an adolescent boy who has been scheduled for an inguinal herniorrhaphy. Both by verbal expressions and body language, the boy indicates a high level of anxiety about the surgery. The young, kindly surgeon who is caring for the adolescent is busy writing in the chart, and completely fails to observe the boy's expression of anxiety. When the boy insists that he is nervous and fears the operation, the surgeon gives him a blanket kind of reassurance. When the boy asks about what is going to happen to him, the surgeon misguidedly tells him not to worry, and that he will be asleep. When the boy asks other questions, the surgeon again tells him that he has nothing to worry about. The doctor fails to explore the two main concerns of this young man, one of which was that he had heard that people bleed to death during surgery, and another (which was less clearly expressed) dealt with the fact that an inguinal herniorrhaphy was threatening because of the proximity to the sexual organs.

The last example is of a poignant interaction of a young black woman who has a brain tumor with her also-young black physician. This insightful professional is not put off by the teen's cheerful, flippant behavior. He manages to break through the young woman's defensive posture and help her express both her fears and feelings of depression about the tumor from which she is suffering.

Assigning Responsibility for Improving Communications

I hope that two main points come through this discussion of our research over the years. One of these points is that effective physician-patient communication is not just a matter of personality, good intentions, and the "art of medicine." Instead, effective communication depends on a number of factors which are researchable. Since the elements of communication are researchable, I also believe that communication is therefore a topic which is very teachable.

The second point which I would stress — and I cannot stress it enough — is that I do not believe we should put the entire burden of improving the communication process on children and families. Some of the presentations at this Round Table have suggested that parents and children should assume some of this responsibility, and that is probably not completely inappropriate — as long as the "some" is emphasized.

The point is that I think that health professionals must assume a major portion of the responsibility for communicating with parents and children. Although many people seem to despair because health professionals are not reaching out effectively, I have *not* given up on them. It seems to me that there are two ways to respond to professionals' lack of effective communication. One way is to plan around the professionals, and the other is to stick with them and keep working to make them effective communicators. This is the course that I, for one, hope we will all pursue.

In brief summary then, this discussion highlights the importance of health professionals (specifically physicians, in this case) reaching out to patients, attempting to get on the wave length of patients, and accepting patients' value systems, concerns, perceptions of their illness, emotions, and feelings. These efforts are essential to establishment of a therapeutic alliance. Findings from our research as well as the case illustrations indicate that attention to the patient as a person with feelings, ideas, and an idiosyncratic background — although at times appearing to be time-consuming — in effect makes for more effective doctor-patient communication and better cooperation for medical treatment.

DISCUSSION

Lee Schorr: Would you tell us a little more about your efforts to use what you have learned from research? Have you applied it in residency training and postgraduate education?

Barbara Korsch: We have applied it beginning with first-year medical students, which, of course, is when it is best received. And we have taught communication skills through all four years of medical school, in house office training, in fellowship training, and with graduate physicians. If you ask how well the training worked, my quantitative data certainly are rather poor. For example, once we gave house officers a lot of experience with playback of videotapes and so on, and did a validation study. We got greatly increased patient satisfaction, and we had anecdotal evidence that the house officers had incorporated some of the desired communication behavior. Unfortunately, the study was not well controlled, for it lasted a couple of years, and other things were changing. The study happened to come at a time when there began to be changes in health professionals themselves; they were becoming more humanitarian and more aware of patients' needs. At about this same time, patients began to be more aware of their own rights, had more knowledge of their own bodies, and made more demands. So I certainly do not want to take credit for what was quite a dramatic change in practice in that setting, although if you saw patient-physician interactions before and after we provided training, I think you would probably believe as we did that some improvements came about because of our efforts.

We have also conducted communication training programs for house officers which have been discouraging from the point of view of demonstrable change in communication skills. However, as you know, there are many factors in house officer training which are counter-productive to teaching communications. So when you look at the very small amount of time that we were given, maybe the results were not as bad as I felt at times they were. Regarding efforts with graduate physicians, we have no representative samples.

Yet, despite the lack of hard data regarding the effectiveness of our training, I certainly feel that using the information from our original research is very effective in teaching professionals. It is interestingly amusing. The professionals do not go to sleep because the information is specific. It is talking to them in a mode that they can accept because it works through the head and not through the heart. At one time I worked with some people who were trying to introduce psychological principles into pediatrics, and they were always making health professionals feel that they had to be better people. The message was that the professionals had to be more patient and understanding, and that they had to take more time. All these are very unwelcome messages to the busy health professional. So we have tried to teach professionals to work smarter, not harder. As those of you who have read about our work know, most of the things we talk about do not involve a tremendous extra expenditure of time or money. So it has been much more fun teaching with our research data as a background, and I think that the recipients have enjoyed it more. How effective the training has been, however, is obviously a big, big question.

Bob Chamberlin: Barbara, I guess that after 15 years of trying to improve the way physicians communicate and conduct well child care, my feeling is essentially that it is too expensive and that there are other people who do it a lot better. Therefore, I would supplement the physician with other people to do most of the well child care. I would agree that you need to concentrate on better communication with sick child care, but I think other professionals do it a lot better in well child care. Would you disagree with that?

Barbara Korsch: I guess so, although I'm on very shaky grounds. I do not doubt there are many other people who can take care of well children very effectively. But I do not think, from our observations, that anyone can quite take the place of the physician. I think there is something about the physician's role which makes the doctor's health communication more powerful minute-for-minute than is true for other health professionals. I think this is more apt to be the case in sick child care than in well child care, but I think that the physician can get away with certain things that others cannot. For example, the physician can get away with fairly direct inquiry and with giving fairly direct advice, and sometimes that's not all bad. I am thinking, for instance, about David Levy, who was one of my earliest teachers, and who wrote an article a long time ago called *The Psychiatric Physical Examination.* (*Editors' note:* See Korsch, *Practical Techniques of Observing Interviewing,* 1956.) It was marvelous because he pointed out how a physician, while conducting a physical examination, can ask patients about certain features of their functioning and about how they compare themselves to others. While there are others who can do physicals, there is something about the doctor-patient relationship that is special. For example, nurses can do physicals, but they have other attitudes which physicians do not have; it is more comfortable for them to listen and to be nondirective. So I think each profession has something different to contribute.

Bob Pantell: I want to say that I agree with some of your emphasis on training physicians. A lot of the work you have done shows that physicians initiate most of the interactions during any type of interview, whether it is a well child or acute visit. Therefore, I think it is up to them to control the direction of the interview. While I think it is interesting that you, along with others, have been able to actually improve physicians' interviewing behaviors, what has always fascinated me has been research which shows that medical students' interview-taking abilities decline. They start out being able to elicit underlying concerns and being psychosocially oriented, but as they go through medical school they become more and more focused on the "classic medical interview." The point is, basically, that medical education has taken away some good communication skills, and now some of us are trying to give them back.

I think physician satisfaction is another important element which you didn't look at, but which some of us in training programs are concerned with because we see a lot of unhappy house officers. We see a lot of primary care physicians burning out, and I think that unless physicians start to learn some of the more imaginative perceptions of what causes symptoms, and so on, they will tend to get bored. So I think there are real benefits besides patient benefits to teaching communication skills to physicians.

Barbara Korsch: I couldn't agree with you more, and I would like to take that point one step further. I think there are other physician needs which we have not mentioned here that are not being met. I think that professionals in training are not being helped to deal with a great many of the overwhelming issues they face in medical care. These include patients' pain, death, dying, chronic illness, hostility, and dependency. These are very, very hard to take if you are expected to deal with them day after day. So besides teaching communication skills, I think we also have to help physicians deal with suffering and emotions.

Lee Schorr: How do you reconcile the point you just made with what you said earlier about teaching through the head and not through the heart?

Barbara Korsch: Dealing with suffering and emotion does get closer to the heart and is much tougher to teach, but I think it also needs attention. You can teach through the head about not withdrawing, not being devastated yourself, not being so hurt that you do not want to hear any more. I think it helps to make these legitimate and conscious areas of inquiry and discussion, because most health professionals are made to feel that they have to be some sort of super people who do not suffer, who do not have negative feelings, and who can handle everything unendingly. Even intellectual awareness helps prevent physicians' feelings of inadequacy.

Bill Frankenburg: If you had to do it over again, I wonder whether you might start out by training your faculty first. The reason I ask is that I think that department chairmen set the tone and everyone else follows through. I am wondering whether perhaps some faculty members' tone is set by their department chairmen, who seem to me very biologically- and disease-oriented.

Barbara Korsch: I think both selection and training of faculty are essential, especially in many tertiary care settings, where the models who are the heroes are people who are absolutely on the low end of the spectrum as far as communication skills are concerned. They are the highly technological specialists who measure their achievement on a very different scale. I have always felt that most of the technological faculty which constitutes models for our residents are not burned out. I think they essentially have never burned out, for they chose their speciality or their way of practicing because they did not want to engage in supportive communication. Since that is what the young doctors are exposed to, they get very little feedback or encouragement for communicating effectively. I guess if I had unlimited sums of money to spend, I would probably train faculty before I would train residents. The trouble is that you get faculty members very late, when it is harder to change their attitudes and behavior.

THE DEVELOPMENT OF CONCEPTS ABOUT ILLNESS

Ellen C. Perrin, M.D.

The idea that children's thinking develops through a series of levels of understanding is based on Piaget's concept of the child as a philosopher, whose work is to make the universe intelligible. Children collect data both from their own observations and from the people they care for around them, and plug the new information into the unfinished puzzle which is their existing set of concepts. Thus, development of understanding about a particular area — illness, for example — depends on getting *correct* information, and getting it in a way that makes sense for the child's current cognitive level. The best way to know what a particular child's concepts are about a phenomenon is to ask, but having a general framework of understanding of the *typical* stages of children's concept development is helpful in knowing where to start.

The sequence of stages in the development of children's understanding of illness has been quite well delineated, while their understanding of how the body works has been somewhat less well described. However, since I think the two are intimately connected, I will try to outline briefly what we know in both of these areas.

Children's Understanding of the Body

Children in the preschool period generally think more empirically than logically, and don't have much sense of causality. They simply take events and things which are contiguous in time and place to be cause and effect, which partly explains why their logic often seems so circular (for example, "Night comes so we can go to sleep," and "Trees grow so we can eat fruit"). Young children are also very egocentric, and say things like, "I can't see Mary's dreams because she doesn't want me to."

Young children must see things to believe that they exist; if something can't be seen, they simply make up an analogy with other things that they *have* seen. This is the origin of the magical thinking which is so typical of preschoolers; they believe that they are very powerful, and that their thoughts and wishes can make all sorts of things happen.

Preschoolers' notions of how the body works are as oversimplified and magical as you might expect — actually even more so, we've found, presumably because there are so few direct ways to discover what's inside the body or how it works. Children of this age also tend to be very anthropomorphic, and just as they may say that cows moo "because they don't want to talk people-talk," they also explain parts of their bodies as having intentions and autonomous desires. The heart and lungs are typically conceptualized as one unit by children up to seven or eight years of age, and their relationship is usually very confused. For example, the heart "makes you breathe by pumping air in and out," or, "The air you breathe pushes your heart and makes it pump." Only around age seven do children understand the heart as pushing blood through the body, and not until age eight or nine do they offer any theory as to *how* or *why* it fulfills this function. The brain is seen by preschoolers as static and unidimensional; a preschooler might say that the brain "makes you think." There would be no explanation as to how it "makes you think" — it just does. A child this age might say that if you didn't have a brain, you'd be "stupid" or "you couldn't think right."

Children's understanding of the function of blood is similarly fascinating. As I have pointed out, preschool and early elementary-age children believe what they see. As a result, even very young children, when asked what's in the body, typically mention blood and the skin — because these are among the few things the children are likely to have seen. When the topic is pursued with children of this age, it becomes clear that they imagine the body to be very like a big plastic bag filled with red liquid which simply sloshes around. When asked what would a person be like without skin, children below about seven years usually respond, "They'd be gross," or, "You'd shrivel up." But when asked what the blood *does* in the body, young children are bewildered; they say things like, "Nothing, it's just there," or, "It's so you'll know when you get hurt." One six-year-old told me, "If you didn't have blood then something else would have to come out when you get cut."

As children get a little older, they begin to understand interrelationships between parts or events, as well as transformations (the process of change from one entity to another through an active process). At around nine or 10 years of age, children understand that some parts of the body are connected and interdependent, and they can talk about some of the active processes which go on inside the body. The children still think very concretely, however, and they solve theoretical problems based on observable objects and events. It's not until the early teen-age years that children typically explain the heart's function as "to pump the blood all around your body" and the brain's as "to tell you what to do" or "to control your senses." What they don't see until much later is the interrelationship of the heart, blood, lungs, brain, and so on, and the notion of the many active processes within the body in which all parts have a functional share.

Children's Understanding of Illness

The early literature regarding children's understanding of illness focused on two themes. The first was the emotional impact of hospitalization and illness, and the other was the recurring theme of illness as punishment (or at least as the expected result of not obeying the rules). Though each of these themes is related to children's conceptual understanding of illness mechanisms, the cognitive development of illness concepts has been clarified only recently. Because the development of these concepts seems to be different in healthy children from that of hospitalized children or children with a chronic illness, I will describe first what we know best, which are the stages healthy children go through.

A couple of early studies pointed out that it was only after 10 to 12 years of age that children began to understand illness as a complex, multifaceted process caused by the interrelationships of many host and agent factors.

More recently, Bibace and Walsh outlined a developmental progression in how children understand the causes of illness. This progression begins with the stages of "phenomenism" (in which the child sees the cause of illness as an external phenomenon which occurs coincident with the illness) and "contagion" (in which the child sees the cause of illness as a concrete agent which is located in nearby objects or people). These stages are typical of children in the preoperational stage, mostly below seven years of age. Children seven to 10 years old are described as being in the stage of "contamination," or — later — "internalization." In these stages, Bibace and Walsh believe that the child understands illness as caused by a "bad" person, object, or external event; this "badness" becomes harmful through some sort of physical contact or through ingestion or inhalation. Children of 12 or over, who are capable of formal operational thinking, can give so-called physiological explanations of illness causation, in which they see the cause of illness as being within the body. Bibace and Walsh explain this sequence of understanding illness by noting the increasing differentiation between self and other which children are able to make as they grow in cognitive sophistication.

In our studies, we have seen a similar progression of understanding of illness, although we have approached the topic using a slightly broader framework. We, too, have based our investigations on a Piagetian model of cognitive development. But we are impressed to find that in addition to children's increasing differentiations of self and other, they also develop increasing sophistication in understanding several other important concepts. These concepts include multiple causation (that multiple things may be associated with causing an event), transformation (that phenomena may undergo qualitative changes from one entity to another), identity (that despite observable changes, objects maintain their basic structure), and relativity (that events and objects don't always follow an invariant pattern but depend on other events or circumstances). It seems to us that as these concepts develop, children have increased ability to understand the complexity of illness causation, and also the prevention and treatment of illness.

Understanding of Illness in Preschool Children

As I mentioned earlier in this paper, children functioning at a preoperational stage of cognitive development characteristically are mainly aware of immediate experiences and those which are easily understood. At this age, children don't differentiate well between the essential features of an event or object and features which are coincidental. For example, they may think that a boat floats "because it's red" or "because it's big"; that is, since color and size are the boat's most outstanding features, they must explain the phenomenon of floating. Young children cannot understand processes and mechanisms because they focus on a single aspect of experiences or objects, without reference to the whole phenomenon and without generalizing from isolated observations.

With regard to illness, this means that young children — up to age six at least — tend to define illness only when they are told that they are ill. They believe that sickness is caused by some concrete action and they think they can avoid illness by obeying a set of rigid rules (such as, "Eat right," "Don't drink out of someone else's glass," "Wear a warm jacket," and, "Stay away from sick people"). Although they believe in such rules, young children can't explain why or how these rules prevent illness. Similarly, young children expect to recover from illness either automatically or by rigidly adhering to another set of rules (such as staying in bed and drinking chicken soup).

Children at this age think that if a certain specific event occurs, the consequences are sure to be seen in a specific outcome. They do not understand that a coincidence of several events, or an interrelationship of external events and internal states, might cause or cure illness. Young children cannot explain, for example, why once going out in the rain without boots was followed by an upper respiratory illness but another time it was not, or why *they* got a rash but their brother did not. Although they cannot explain these phenomena, they are not concerned, for they believe in the existence and power of magic! They don't need to explain any *mechanism* by which the agents they identify cause, prevent, or cure disease: they just do. This circular reasoning was demonstrated by a six-year-old with asthma who told us that "you get asthma from breathing too fast." A seven-year-old responded to the question, "How can you get better if you have an asthma attack?" with, "Don't wheeze." Interestingly, these children also typically respond to the question, "When you aren't sick, what are you?" with, "I'm just myself," or, "I'm Bobby" — as if illness is something entirely outside of and separate from themselves.

Understanding of Illness by Eight- to Ten-Year-Olds

By eight to 10 years of age, children are likely to apply the logic of concrete operational thinking to their understanding of illness. They are fascinated by classifying and categorizing, and they are bound by rigid rules; for a child of this age, there are rarely two "right" answers or two ways to do something. Thus, children at this stage usually define illness by a set of multiple concrete symptoms, and they do not generalize from these symptoms to others. They believe that illnesses are caused only or primarily by germs, although they usually can offer no explanation of how the germs make a person sick. Typically, children of this age expect to recover from illness by "taking care of themselves" and allowing medicines and "whatever the doctor says" to act on the illness. Because of this thinking, eight- to 10-year-olds are likely to be passive about health care; they see outside factors as both causing and curing illness, and have only a limited understanding of how the body heals itself. Thus, to keep healthy, simply, "Don't go anywhere near sick people." They still do not understand the mechanisms of illness, although they are beginning to be able to explain complex mechanisms of physical causality (such as how a bicycle works or how night comes).

Understanding of Illness by Older Children

The ideas that healthy 10- to 12-year-olds express about illness are more sophisticated. In fact, around age 11 or 12 there is a remarkable jump in the sophistication of children's concepts about illness. By this age, children no longer believe that the mere existence of things or events is sufficient to cause, treat, or prevent illness. They see that things and events actively interact to affect health. In addition, they are beginning to understand that germs cause illnesses by entering the body and "using up the vitamins and stuff you need." As a child of this age might explain, "Things you're allergic to don't *always* make you have an asthma attack. You have to get them inside your body and they have to do something in there." Similarly, medicines are seen to work by doing something active inside the body (for example, medicine might "kill the germs" or "dissolve the stuff in your lungs").

By the time children reach the formal operational stage described by Piaget, they are able to think hypothetically, filling gaps in their knowledge with generalizations from prior experiences. They can understand illness in terms of internal structures and systems whose dysfunction can be revealed by a variety of external symptoms. Typically, older children define illness in abstract terms with an emphasis on internal feelings of non-wellness, independent of specific complaints or external signs. These children answer the question, "How do children know when they're sick?" with responses like, "You just don't feel right."

They typically also understand that there are many interrelated causes of illness, that the body may respond variably to one or a combination of agents, and that illness is both caused and cured as a result of a complex interaction between host and agent factors. Their explanations of how medicine works reveal that they know that the body's response is critical if a medication is to be effective, and that it is the body itself that must "defeat the germs."

Prevention of illness is apparently a more difficult concept to grasp than are causation and treatment. Even by age 13, very few healthy children seem to understand prevention in any more abstract terms than typical 10- to 12-year-olds.

Chronically Ill Children's Understanding of Illness

Children with chronic illness have considerably more experience than healthy children with the causes and treatment of illness, and the prevention of complications. Therefore, we have wondered if chronically ill children would have a more sophisticated understanding of illness. Our preliminary evidence suggests that children with diabetes or asthma do indeed have a somewhat more sophisticated understanding of illness concepts at all ages. While healthy children show a marked increase in their understanding at around 11 or 12 years, children with asthma or diabetes demonstrate this spurt around nine years. These differences are especially marked in specific content areas. Children with diabetes, for example, seem to understand prevention better than healthy children; children with asthma are more sophisticated in their understanding of the causes of illness. This increased sophistication probably directly reflects the important management issues which children with these two diseases face each day.

We were surprised to find that chronically ill children understood the mechanisms involved in their own illness at a less sophisticated level than the way they understood the mechanisms of causation, prevention, and treatment of illness in general. This was especially true of children below the age of 12.

Professionals' Awareness of Children's Understanding of Illness

We did a small survey to assess how well professionals know what to expect from children in the realm of illness concepts. Not surprisingly, we found they do not know much. What's interesting is the *pattern* of professionals' misunderstanding of children's concepts. Both nurses and physicians estimate the age of children's statements best in the seven- to 10-year-old group, and in general they overestimate what younger children understand and underestimate what older children understand. We don't really know what professionals actually say to children of various ages, but by extrapolating from our data, we guess that professionals tend to talk to preschool children using vocabulary which is much too advanced. In addition, we think that professionals assume a level of conceptual understanding which is way over children's heads as well. For example, no matter how short the words and how concrete the example, a preschooler cannot understand how oral medication could make sense for a rash, or why he or she should take medicines when not sick; nor would young children understand an explanation of how their bodies' own reactions to a foreign agent cause a number of symptoms.

When a very bright six-year-old was asked, "How do children get sick?" she said, "I think it's the devil. My mom doesn't believe in the devil but I sort of do. I dream about him. I think that the devil sends out little insects that you can't see. The devil can see them — they're great big to him. And they go and search and search and when they see a person they go 'zip' in their mouth. Then, whatever kind of a bug it is you get that sickness — like if it's a 'can't move' bug then you can't move." Later, when asked how children recover from an illness, this girl said, "Get lots of rest." When asked further how resting would help, she said, "When you rest you yawn, and when you yawn the bug can fly back out and then it gets in someone else."

DISCUSSION

Bob Chamberlin: How does your knowledge of how children understand the body and illness influence how you deliver services to children who are chronically ill?

Ellen Perrin: We talk to children differently. And we are starting to put together some intervention programs which involve groups of children of similar ages, or at least in similar stages of development. Basically, we are trying to give children usable information in a conceptual framework they understand. For example, we are putting together groups of children with asthma and diabetes, and giving them specific explanations of what their illness is all about. I find it remarkable how little they have understood. Even the children who have had diabetes for years and who have known the right things to say when the doctors or nurses asked them what was happening, have not understood the internal mechanisms involved.

Bob Pantell: I think it is very easy for children to make physicians think they are more sophisticated than they really are. Children have very good memories, and they are very good at repeating information. So I often see asthmatic children go into lengthy explanations or use large words that they have heard from others. They say, "I've got these triggers that set my asthma attacks off." If you ask what they mean, they say, "The triggers inside just go off." I think health professionals need to be careful not only about thinking children are more sophisticated than they really are. I think professionals also must be careful about the imagery they use with children. For example, we were seeing a boy last week for chronic abdominal pain, and took a series of x-rays. One professional showed the child the x-ray and said, "Gee, look at that! It looks like a flying saucer." As a result, the child thought he had aliens in his stomach who were trying to drill their way out.

Earl Schaefer: When you talk about mental age and chronological age, does mental age make a difference? I find that many low-income parents conceptualize their child's behavior very differently from how the teacher conceptualizes the child's behavior. I wonder whether we can generalize that if people are less well educated or from a lower socioeconomic group, maybe their conceptual schemes are different.

Ellen Perrin: The children on which our initial interviews were done were very bright. They were children with mean IQs of 120, and I suspect that had we interviewed children with a more average IQ, our results would have come out slightly different. I think the sequence of understanding is the same, regardless of IQ, but I am not sure about the exact age levels at which you would see different areas of understanding.

Bill Frankenburg: I have a question about an issue you did not discuss — that of guilt. To what extent do children who have an illness, particularly a chronic illness or disability, feel guilty? Do they feel that they have done something that has caused them to have an illness?

Ellen Perrin: There is a lot of literature which implies that children indeed do feel guilt, especially before the age of 10. My sense is that researchers may have misinterpreted what the children actually said. I don't think they were saying they were sick because they had been bad, but that they were sick because they had not obeyed the rules. It's a fine distinction, but an important one.

Andy Selig: What are the relationships between parents' concepts of the illness and children's concepts of the illness? Is there anything to be said for enhancing children's understanding of illness by working with parents, as opposed to working directly with the children?

Ellen Perrin: All the time I have been doing interviews with children, I have always wanted to talk to the parents and find out what they understood. But we have never done that, and as far as I know, no one else has either. So we do not know what the "adult" norm is in terms of understanding of illness, although I think we all share Evan's feeling that many adults are not all that sophisticated either.

COMMUNICATING WITH CHILDREN IN THE HOSPITAL

Robert H. Pantell, M.D.
and Catherine C. Lewis, Ph.D.

Each year one out of 18 children will leave the familiar surroundings of their homes and neighborhoods, the networks and games of their friends, and the support and care of their parents to enter a foreign and often frightening social system and institution — the hospital. In this strange and unusual environment, the child is not only required to recover from an illness, but to demonstrate good citizenship as well. These expectations are — to say the least — a tall order for a sick six-year-old. (By way of contrast, consider the amount of orientation that medical students have by the time they become interns, and recall the amount of anxiety and emotional upset that they experience as they are required to assume a new role in the hospital.)

Research makes clear that there are numerous psychological consequences of a hospital stay for children. While most hospitalizations are transient, there are some associations between early and prolonged or repeated hospitalizations and behavioral disturbances in adolescents (Table 1). In contrast, as the table shows, some children may also have positive responses to hospitalization. This is more likely to be true for eight- to 11-year-olds than for either younger or older children. What is clear is that the way a child experiences a hospital stay and what a child learns from this experience can be influenced by medical professionals. The purpose of this paper is to review some of the existing theories and research focusing on hospitalized children, and to develop a conceptual framework and practical guidelines for communicating with these children.

Table 1. Consequences of Hospitalization

I. During Hospitalization

Anxiety
- Separation
- Mutilation
- Physiology: heart rate, blood pressure, sweat, muscle, voiding, emesis
- Loss of control
- Pain
- Death

Behavior
- Crying
- Cooperation
- Motor activity
- Anesthesia induction

Psychologic Disturbance
- Hysterical conversion reaction
- Depression
- Psychosis

II. Immediately After Hospitalization

Regression
- Immature behavior: thumb sucking, enuresis, encopresis, baby talk, clinging, crying, eating
- Increased dependency
- Decreased attention span

Sleep

Anxiety
- Won't leave home
- Fear of doctors/nurses

Aggression

Progression
- Self-esteem
- Accelerated learning

III. Years After Hospitalization

Behavior
- Disturbance
- Delinquency
- Unstable job pattern
- Poor reading

Because of this, communication with hospitalized children is more than a social amenity; it is important therapeutically. In fact, a variety of studies have demonstrated that such communication can reduce anxiety prior to hospitalization, can improve behavior during the hospital stay, and can promote psychological adjustment after discharge. Physiologic parameters have also been influenced by communication, as have medication requests and lengths of stay. The evidence for communicating with children to reduce the psychological burdens of hospitalization is shown in Table 2.

Preparing Children for Hospitalization

Many studies have shown the benefits of preparing children for hospitalization. The goals of such preparations are to help children adjust to hospitalization and to make it a less frightening experience. This is accomplished by: providing the child with information; allowing the child emotional expression; establishing a relationship with

Table 2. Experimental Studies on Hospitalized Children

Intervention	Conditions	Outcomes
Puppet therapy	Cardiac catheterization	Behavior
Coloring book	Tonsillectomy	Anxiety
Parent support	Elective surgery	Psychologic measures
Child support	Anesthesia induction	Parent satisfaction
Home preparation		Parent calls
Hospital preparation		Post-discharge behaviors
Stress-point preparation		Progression
Film modeling		

the child; probing the child's and family's explanatory models; encouraging the child to practice scheduled medical procedures; and describing what the child will experience.

Children have many frightening misconceptions of what goes on in the hospital. These misconceptions arise from many factors. For example, developmental level may be involved (younger children fear punishment is the cause for hospitalization and worry about abandonment and mutilation). Personal experience impacts a child's understanding (this may include births and deaths). Other factors include fantasies and the media (which may resemble reality less than a child's fantasies). The importance of the media and of books should not be underrated. Children are exposed to many television programs and movies in which the players (both patients and staff) have humerous interchanges (punctuated with electronic laughs) or act heroically. Even some children's books portray ever-smiling staff, with doctors walking children hand-in-hand to the operating room. The point is that children need realistic expectations of what will occur in the hospital.

Other problems can arise because parents often expect their children to be "model patients" and reflect well on their families. Parents and children should be given permission for their children to both feel and act sick, and should know that letting the child adopt the sick role behavior for a short period of time is acceptable. Parents and children should also be encouraged to express their feelings about what is to occur as well as their concerns, questions, and apprehensions. This will give the health professional an opportunity to correct misconceptions, convey realistic expectations, and acknowledge feelings of anxiety, fear, and sadness. Despite the advantages, this communication process has several pitfalls. For example, communication may be difficult because parents may lack knowledge of the procedures and children's experiences may be limited. Medical professionals may also have several limitations, including limited ability to convey this type of information, limited skill in eliciting concerns and providing support, limited experience in coping with uncertainty, and limited ability to accurately convey the risks and benefits of various procedures.

There are many ways of accomplishing the goals of preparing children and their families for hospitalization. For example, many hospitals have prehospitalization programs directed by child-life workers, social workers, or nurses. These programs have the advantage of allowing children and their families to become familiar with hospital surroundings. Some physicians use an office visit for preparation; numerous educational films and books are available for this purpose, but these should always be used as "triggers" to encourage a child's active participation in the process.

The timing of preparation is also important, and the child's age is a key variable. Younger children may have difficulties with memory if prepared for hospitalization too far in advance, while older children should not have to ponder for too many days their coming "ordeal." For a routine hospitalization, preparation several days in advance is generally advised. While many hospitalizations are acute, eliminating the possibility of a formal preparation program, the goals are the same and should be accomplished by staff and for parents as soon after the admission as possible.

The Benefits of Preparation

As has been already mentioned, we have conducted a number of studies which have demonstrated that formal preparation procedures for children result in improved outcomes during and after hospitalization (Table 2). Preparations directed to parents are grounded in social interaction theory, which states that reduction in anxiety to parents will indirectly benefit children. This has been upheld in the studies of Skipper and Leonard and Visintainer and Wolfer. Studies of children who view films depicting other children successfully coping with a stressful event are based on Bandura and Menlove's work showing that such modeling can reduce anxiety-motivated avoidance behavior. The child-model displays anxiety, but successfully completes the task without adverse consequences. Since moderate physiologic and emotional arousal also increases imitation of a model, a child's anxiety while viewing a modeling film may facilitate attention and foster learning.

Several studies have looked at particular elements used in preparation, including the type of information, use of films, and primary emotional support. Other studies have examined the usefulness of combined preparation approaches. For example, Wolfer and Visintainer offered parents and children both information and opportunities to explore feelings before surgery; experimental group children had better recovery of physiologic parameters (heart rate, fluid intake, voiding) and evidenced less upset, a higher degree of cooperation, and better post-hospital adjustment than the control group. These researchers also demonstrated the effectiveness of a home program in which children used information and procedures employed in previous preparation studies.

While these studies are encouraging and offer principles and guidelines for communicating with children, they are limited in that they have been conducted exclusively on children experiencing routine and standardized procedures.

Communication in the Hospital

The goals of communication are similar whether in a formal preparation session or a bedside chat once the child is hospitalized. During the hospital stay, it is important for professionals to give children as much control as possible for their new environment. Communication with children can be envisioned in Figure 1.

Much of the communication about illness is funneled through parents, which is appropriate for younger children. However, our studies indicate that while physicians solicit a great amount of information from children, they provide information primarily to parents. Health professionals should be aware of this paradoxical model, for we are concerned that it may create a passive role for children.

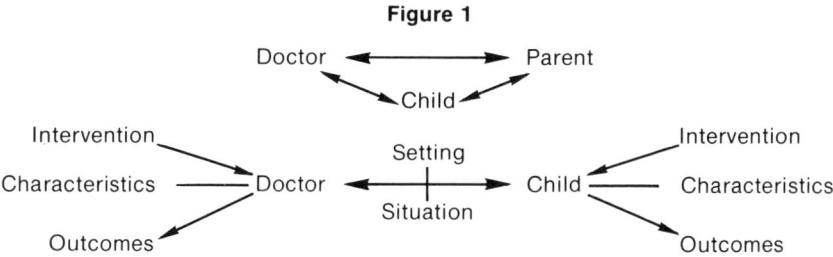

Figure 1

Child Characteristics

Cognitive ability. Substantial research shows that the most important aspects of a child's ability to interpret and participate in the illness process is the child's age or cognitive level. What adults say about hospitalization and what children hear may be very different. for children shape information about disease and about medical procedures so that it fits their own concepts. A rapidly growing body of research shows that children's concepts of health, illness, bodily functions, and medical procedures change systematically with age, following a course similar to other cognitive concepts. Thus, a four-year-old may believe that repeated blood tests permanently deplete the blood supply and cause death by draining. A seven-year-old may believe that exposure to any disease automatically results in illness. In their early years, children frequently view illness as punishment or as magically contagious. Later, children learn the role of external agents, such as germs. Finally, children learn the role of internal factors such as genetic traits, and they learn of the interaction between external and internal factors. But even by the eighth grade, less than half of all children demonstrate awareness that internal and external factors interact to produce disease.

Children's concepts of the body's interior also seem to undergo change with age. When children of six or seven draw a picture of the interior of the human body, it typically contains a few organs which are perceptible from the outside (such as the bones and the beating heart) and some free-floating substances the child has witnessed entering or leaving the body (food, blood, and feces). As they grow older, children learn that food and other ingested substances are housed in various internal organs, that these organs can have more than one function, and that they work in close coordination.

Children's concepts of medical procedures may also show dramatic developmental change. The young child, not skilled in role-taking, may believe that physicians cannot know that a procedure is painful unless the child cries out. Young children's thoughts tend to be concrete and static. Therefore, focusing on the needle and its attendant pain, children may refuse to believe that there is medicine inside a syringe and that it is transferred to the child's own body.

Recent research does not suggest that there are hard-and-fast age-related stages in children's concepts in these various domains. Children's reasoning levels differ across diseases, and each level of reasoning shows a great age spread. The research does demonstrate that children assimilate what they hear about disease to fit their own concepts. Health professionals must know something about those concepts before they can assess the impact of their own words on the child. Health professionals may also be able to help children along to more sophisticated levels of reasoning. While there is no experimental evidence on this point, there is evidence that young children who know about the role of germs in transmitting disease are less likely to believe that illness is punishment.

Table 3. Communicating with Hospitalized Children

Ages 0–3

1. Allow child prior, non-stressful exposure to new perceptual experiences: lights, masks, uniforms, smells, restraints
2. Allow child to establish sense of control by handling equipment, performing procedures on dolls
3. Provide parent information and allow expression of concerns
4. Assure child return of parents

Ages 4–7

1. Provide child with models of coping responses
2. Allow child to rehearse coping responses to painful/stressful procedure
3. Help child distinguish attainable goals: blood tests cannot be avoided, but can be shortened by child's action
4. Explore concepts of illness, hospitalization and procedures

   Misconceptions include:
   a. Illness and procedures are punishment
   b. Do not believe what can't be seen, e.g., spots only caused externally
   c. Lumping organ systems: the heart pumps when you breathe
   d. Blood is a fixed quantity which can be permanently depleted
   e. All diseases are contagious
   f. Procedures which hurt aren't therapeutic
5. Explore concerns about separation, mutilation, physical pain, guilt

Ages 8–12

1. Explore concerns about impact on peer relations, especially sense of inferiority
2. Explore illness concepts

   Misconceptions include:
   a. Inability to consider simultaneously numerous causes or factors in disease
   b. Failure to recognize changes in mood, motivation, state, and role accompanying illness
   c. Failure to understand interdependency among organ systems
   d. No awareness of preventive actions
3. Egocentric thinking: Doctor doesn't know procedure is painful unless you cry

Ages 13–18

1. Explore concerns about body image, independence, sexual identity, interference with ability to establish identity especially likely
2. Tendency to deny or minimize severity of illness
3. May desire more information about etiology and prognosis than physician provides

Table 3 summarizes our recommendations for age-appropriate communication with children.

Sex. Considerable work has evaluated the role of a child's sex on reactions to hospitalization. Mechanic showed that boys were raised to be more stoic about illness than girls. Our group has documented the fact that physicians interact differently with boys by giving them more information.

Personality. Although the literature linking prehospitalization personality with hospital adjustment is far from conclusive, it appears that well-adjusted, intelligent children who have good relationships with their parents may be less prone to upset. Other important background variables include previous hospitalizations, previous separations, recent life events, length of illness, and severity of the problem.

It is important to focus briefly on how children cope with the hospital. Beuf has developed an interesting classification system. She lists five patterns which are not necessarily mutually exclusive: the wild kid, the gregarious host, embracing the sick role, the junior medical student (taking on the characteristics of oppressors), and withdrawal. (The last role is a particular problem for health professionals, for it is essentially the role of learned helplessness.)

This and other discussions of children's characteristics have focused on what the children are capable of understanding. What they actually *want* to know is a different question. In general, children are interested in the immediate events that will affect their lives. The time they must go to x-ray today is usually more important to children than the results of yesterday's tests. Parents, of course, tend to be most interested in prognosis. The dilemma for our communication model is that doctors often seem preoccupied with precise diagnostic categorization and are not always capable of translating this to either prognoses or to the time of tomorrow's x-ray. A recent study of adolescents with cancer illustrates this point well. It showed that physicians were not good predictors of adolescents' chief concerns. Physicians thought adolescents would be most interested in how they could help with the treatment, including calling the doctor, and in the long-term effects of treatment on their appearances. Instead, adolescents were found to be most interested in what to expect if the cancer spread, in the prevention of cancer, and in the results of tests. In general, adolescents were more likely to be interested in some of the technical aspects of their disease than their physicians predicted.

Setting

While the "setting" under discussion in Figure 1 is the hospital, the children exhibit different communication patterns in their own rooms, in hospital playrooms, and in procedure rooms. It is important that hospitals provide "safe" areas for children where they are free to interact without fear of an invasive event.

Situation

The "situation" in our communication model is particularly important, for a hospital has many unique situations. We should like to focus on some practical lessons that can be learned from two of these situations: bedside rounds and invasive procedures.

Bedside rounds have been both advocated and condemned in recent literature. While there are risks of presenting new or confusing data to children and parents in this indirect fashion, bedside rounds also provide an opportunity for families to both witness and participate in the process of care. We are currently conducting a series of investigations examining the impact of open bedside rounds on parents and children.

Invasive procedures are often synonomous with painful procedures. However, pain is a sense which can be modified by a series of distraction techniques or by hypnosis. *(Editors' note:* Here, Dr. Pantell showed a brief videotape which demonstrated distraction techniques performed by a physician during a spinal tap on a school-age boy. The physician acknowledged the boy's fright, distracted the boy by talking about the coming of winter, and encouraged him to actively participate in a conversation by discussing pleasurable events like playing in the snow.)

Intervention

While I have discussed formal preparation for hospitalization, a variety of other interpersonal interventions, activities, and structural alterations may be effective in improving targeted in-hospital outcomes. These include age-appropriate play activities, and respect for the autonomy of the child and family. It is important for professionals to individualize these preparation activities by understanding, for example, that puppet therapy is not a panacea. For an adolescent, an activity which instead involves access to a telephone may have remarkable effects.

Outcomes

While most studies have focused on children's hospital and post-hospital behavioral disturbances as desired outcomes, there are many other outcomes which merit further examination. These include functional status, sense of control, knowledge, satisfaction with health status, and satisfaction with medical care.

Physician Characteristics

Physician characteristics, skills, and training are all important to this discussion, for physicians initiate the majority of communication interactions with children and their families.

The actual communication by the physician is principally dependent on the physician's skill in cognitively appropriate interactions (verbal and play) as well as the established relationship the physician has with the child. One aspect of verbal communication where physicians unfortunately have few skills is in the use of symbols. For a child, application of a Band-aid may symbolize the completion of a test, and biting off the bracelet the end of hospitalization. Aspects of the physician-child/family relationship which are important are the duration of time the physician has been involved with the child/family, the perceived competence of the physician, the physician's consistency and perceived truthfulness, and the physician's perceived technical skills.

The Dilemma of Medical Communication

While this paper has focused on the process of communication, it is appropriate to finish with a comment on the hierarchy and dilemma of medical communication. It is not unreasonable to assume that many of the physicians who care for children in hospitals entered the profession because they liked children. The same can be said of the nurses, child-life workers, and social workers who are employed on pediatric wards. However, many physicians — especially early in training — are forced to assume the role of "bad guys" through repeatedly drawing blood, inserting intravenous needles, and so on. When confronted by the "bad guy" resident, a child may refuse to speak to the intern or answer questions; this may be the only power a child has left in a frightening and painful situation. The intern's plight is made worse when the attending physician takes the limelight during open rounds, demonstrates superior competence, and projects an image of protector of the child. Child-life workers and nurses also find it easier than interns to assume a supportive and nurturing role and encourage the child's expression of feelings. The intern's role is thus made quite precarious in terms of both self-concept and ability to communicate, and — in fact — communication becomes extraordinarily difficult. Thus, it is not surprising that approximately 90 percent of the "medical" communication literature is by non-physicians, nor is it surprising to find that physicians spend only 25 percent of their time interacting with children at the bedside (compared to 50 percent for nurses and 75 percent for child-life workers).

Yet, while the physician's job as a communicator may be difficult, it is not unsurmountable. Knowing what to expect from a child as well as having some interaction skills are the first steps in using communication to establish an ongoing therapeutic relationship with a child.

DISCUSSION

Evan Charney: I would like to raise an organizational issue which relates to the care of children. Looking both at community hospitals and university hospitals, it often is not clear who is in charge of information services or to whom a parent or professional would go to change a system. In many university hospital services, there isn't one person with responsibility for the system. There is a nursing hierarchy, there's a medical hierarchy which changes monthly, there are child-life workers, and there are social services. In community hospitals, it is sometimes better, but it is sometimes worse. In fact, in some community hospitals, no one is in charge. There may be only an elected chief of pediatric services who practices in the community. Yet, community hospitals are where two-thirds of the children in this country are hospitalized. In short, I think we have to pay attention to hospitals' organizational structures if we want to improve communication.

Bob Pantell: I couldn't agree more. I wish our hospitals all had more semblance of a general pediatrician who had some influence on the wards. Unfortunately, most university hospitals are run by different subspecialists. In our hospital, for example, there are about 65 different subspecialists. It is very difficult to deal with issues when so many people are involved. I think what often tends to happen in university hospitals is that subspecialists have the wards organized to meet their needs, and there is no one person in charge who will organize the ward to meet the needs of the child. For example, in one hospital I know of, the thoracic surgeons did not want to walk up another flight of stairs, so they demanded that the adult ICU be placed in the middle of the pediatric floor. This provoked a major fight that literally lasted months and took hundreds of hours on an issue that you would not believe would have to be fought.

Joy Penticuff: Bob, I would like to add just one comment. You made the statement that physicians sometimes feel that they are the "bad guys" in a situation, and I want to respond to that as a nurse. I see how pediatricians could come to that feeling because they write the orders for procedures. But I think that nurses feel that way at times also. Nurses are the ones who give shots and hold the children down for procedures, and who are with the children when their parents leave the units. I think that we are all in this together, and what we must do is to support each other as professionals so that we can be less overwhelmed by some of the difficult aspects of our work with children.

Bob Pantell: I think that is an excellent point.

THE CHILD WITH A CHRONIC ILLNESS

Michael Weitzman, M.D.

Editors' note: Because Dr. Weitzman was unable to be present, his paper was read by Evan Charney, M.D.

Many of the most trying difficulties for those of us who provide services to children with chronic illnesses are related to problems of communication. These problems occur frequently, can be physically and socially damaging, and are often quite difficult to correct. I would like to examine the special communication problems that occur in the care of children who are chronically ill, and to propose some strategies to improve communication.

Communication problems seem to be more common in the care of chronically ill children than in routine health or even acute illness care partly because chronically ill children use many — and many specialized — services. This results in a large number of interactions among the child, family, and professional service providers, and also among professionals. Interprofessional communication is complicated by the need to coordinate services, by difficulties in establishing relationships between multiple individuals, and by tensions that occur when professionals communicate across professional boundaries. Because many of the services that chronically ill children need do not fit neatly into the domain of any particular professional group, there are often both "turf issues" and hazy boundaries of professional responsibility.

Professional-family communication is complicated by a number of factors. First, children with chronic illnesses and their families have very special needs for information and counseling which physicians are often not trained (or accustomed) to provide. Second, parents and children often do not tell medical providers about their expectations or their needs for counseling. Third, because stress markedly decreases cognitive skills, the stress of adapting to a child's chronic illness may alter the communication skills and styles of many children and parents, and may thus interfere with effective communication. Finally, and perhaps most importantly, chronically ill children and their families often experience profoundly disruptive social messages and interactions that directly impact on their self-images and the ways they interact with others.

Communication Problems Arising from the Specialization of Health Services

Many of the communication problems which result in the care of chronically ill children arise from the children's need for highly sophisticated professional services. During the past several decades, medical research and technology have resulted in a dramatic increase in the survival of many children with chronic illnesses. However, an unfortunate and ironic corollary is that the prolonged survival of many of these children has often been accompanied by a set of very complicated physical and psychosocial problems. The complexity of these problems and the technical expertise necessary to address them have resulted in a high degree of specialization, with resulting fragmentation of professional services; this, in turn, has produced interprofessional communication difficulties which often make it very difficult to systematically and effectively meet the needs of chronically ill children.

Comprehensive care for children with chronic illnesses requires that health services meet all the medical and nonmedical health-related needs of the children and their families. Services must therefore be available and organized so that attention is directed to:

1. Problems related to the chronic illness;
2. Medical problems which are not related to the child's chronic illness;

3. Well child and preventive care, including immunizations and screening for disease;
4. Issues of adjustment and adaptation to the illness and its social consequences, including the effects on other family members; and
5. Education and vocational concerns.

Since it is unreasonable to assume that any one person can meet all these needs, the trend has been to rely increasingly on specialists who (formally or informally, for better or for worse) share responsibility for caring for the child and family. General practitioners and pediatricians, pediatric subspecialists, occupational and physical therapists, social and mental health workers, and special educators may all be involved in the care of one child. With such a large array of professionals acting upon and interacting with the child and each other, it is no wonder that certain services are often duplicated and that certain needs go unattended.

Much frustration, dissatisfaction, emotional trauma, and sometimes even suboptimal health care result from communication difficulties that are a consequence of the usual service arrangements for children with chronic illnesses. Although specialists may expertly meet a child's specific needs, certain medical or nonmedical needs of the child may be neglected because of poorly defined or communicated responsibilities and because no one person takes responsibility for overseeing and coordinating all aspects of care. Even in situations where all the care is provided in one institution — such as a medical center or children's hospital — needs may go unmet because of poor coordination and communication. Often one professional attends to one area of care and another to another aspect, but many needs may be overlooked. This is especially true of the child's and family's psychosocial and developmental needs, but it is sometimes also the case for purely medical needs as well.

For example, children with chronic illnesses have the same basic needs for standard well child care as their healthy peers. If no one takes responsibility for monitoring a child's immunization status, it is likely that the child will be inadequately immunized. If no one screens the child for hypertension, anemia, or hearing and vision deficits, these problems are also likely to go undetected.

Similar problems occur when chronically ill children develop acute illnesses. If a child with spina bifida receives care from a variety of physicians, who is responsible for caring for an acute illness? Is it the neurosurgeon, neurologist, urologist, orthopedist, or general pediatrician? Most specialty clinics at medical centers meet only at specified times during the week and are closed on weekends and evenings. If no one is responsible for acute care, or if the family does not know how to reach the appropriate physician, they may have to take the child to an emergency room to be seen by unfamiliar physicians. It can be terribly stressful for parents and children to be dependent on unfamiliar physicians at the very time that the child seems most in need of trusted help. Even medical care may suffer because the acute-care physicians are not familiar with the details of the individual child's problem.

Communication Problems Between Physicians and Other Care Providers

Chronically ill children face a variety of problems because of poor communication between physicians and other health, human services, and education professionals. For example, the input of mental health professionals is often needed by these children and their families, but many physicians are unfamiliar with various psychotherapeutic approaches, and many are skeptical about their utility. Physicians often do not have well-formed networks for mental health referrals, and many are not used to collaborating with mental health workers. In addition there are many mental health agencies which work separately from each other, and many work independently of physicians. These factors often discourage referrals and collaboration, and may result in lack of attention to vital needs.

Comparable problems arise because of poor communication between physicians and school personnel. School is not only the place where children acquire academic skills, it is also where they learn many important interpersonal and social skills. The child who fails in school or who is excluded from school is deprived of many of the experiences that contribute to a lifelong sense of competence and self-worth.

Success in school for children with chronic illnesses often requires collaboration between parents, physicians, and school personnel. Some drugs, such as anti-seizure medications, may make the child drowsy, creating problems with concentration. The school nurse may be reluctant to administer certain drugs on the school premises. School personnel may not know how to manage acute asthma attacks, may not know how to help the child make up missed school work, or may be unsure when the child should be kept home. Physicians can do much to ease these problems by sharing information with school personnel but, unfortunately, physicians often do not routinely collaborate with school personnel. In addition, many parents discourage such communication because they fear if the child's medical condition is known, either preferential or prejudicial treatment will result. In reality, of course, more problems are caused by lack of information than the reverse. Without accurate information, school personnel are forced to make their own interpretations, which are often incorrect and lead to unrealistic and damaging management approaches in the school setting.

Communication Between the Chronically Ill Child, Parents, and Professionals

Noncompliance with treatment recommendations is often a major problem in the long-term management of children with chronic illnesses. Motivating children and families to be actively involved in therapeutic activities, helping them abandon the "sick-role," and normalizing their social experiences as much as possible are often essential to successful medical management and to prevent and correct severe psychosocial maladjustment.

Compliance with treatment recommendations has been shown to be improved by satisfaction with the physician-patient relationship, and by the family's degree of understanding of the disease. Yet numerous studies show that families often lack the information they need if compliance is to be increased. This lack of information is frequently the result of poor communication.

Some communication problems originate with medical personnel, but others originate with the child and family. Anger, guilt, and grief can significantly lessen a family's ability to hear and understand information. Denial is a defense mechanism against stress, and distressful information may have to be repeated again and again if the child and family are to fully understand it. In addition, parents and chronically ill children may be intimidated by professionals, or may take an oppositional stance against the professionals on whom they are most dependent. Other difficulties arise because physicians may be hurried and thus may not take the time to explain details, because physicians may not appreciate the importance of this aspect of care, or because they may be uncomfortable discussing the affect of the illness on the child and family.

Still other communication problems result from the nature of chronic illnesses. Often the medical aspects of the condition are quite complicated, and understanding them requires a fair degree of scientific knowledge. Often the diagnosis or prognosis is uncertain, or the treatment approach highly variable. These factors all can provoke anxiety in the family, and can further decrease satisfaction, understanding, and compliance.

One of the greatest and most frequently overlooked needs of families of children with chronic illnesses is for a consistent, effective exchange of information about the illness, about the limitations the illness imposes, and about the affect the illness has on a family's entire life. Due to misconceptions, unfounded fears, inappropriate expectations, and altered discipline, many children with chronic illnesses develop impaired self-images and behavioral problems which are frequently more disabling than the illness itself. Psychological and social maladjustment are not intrinsic characteristics of chronic childhood illness; rather, they are complications which often result because of lack of information and altered social experiences.

Unfortunately, many health professionals actually contribute to these problems by not addressing them, or by implying (perhaps inadvertently) that they are not important or deserving of professional attention. Rather than viewing the child as an individual with a particular health problem, health care providers frequently define chronically ill children exclusively in terms of their disabilities. This teaches the children to identify with a handicapped role.

Children with chronic illnesses and their families need accurate information concerning realistic expectations, treatment options, and the influence of the illness on such things as child-rearing practices, parental attitudes, social contacts, and family stress. They often need help to lessen anxiety and anger. Knowledge is both a source of a sense of power and a source of power itself, and intellectualization is one of the major defenses for dealing with stress. In addition, knowledge provides the only really useful base for making decisions and eventually coming to terms with an illness. Without accurate information, the child and family are left at the mercy of their imaginations, which is unfortunate because fantasies are often far more terrifying than the truth itself.

Approaches to Improve Communication in the Care of Chronically Ill Children

Although there is no simple solution to the communication problems that occur in the care of chronically ill children, many of the problems could be eased if attention were given to continuity and coordination of services. In most situations, what is needed is reorientation and reorganization of existing services rather than the creation of still more services.

Most professionals and parents of chronically ill children agree on the importance of a satisfying, long-term relationship with one medical provider. As noted earlier, children with chronic illnesses often experience short-term interactions with many professionals. The lack of long-term involvement with an individual physician tends to inhibit the development of a warm, trusting, supportive relationship which leads to effective communication. This often results in parents and children being confused, anxious, and angry because their expectations have not been met. Such experiences can further add to the sense of chaos and alienation which so many of these families experience. In addition, lack of long-term involvement with one health professional may result in lack of attention to psychosocial issues.

Coordination of services is perhaps the most critical element in ensuring quality care for children with chronic illnesses, for lack of such coordination often results in duplication of services or in some needs being unattended. Coordination of services requires that one provider be the focal point in contacts with other providers and agencies. This person directs patients to appropriate specialists, receives feedback from specialists and interprets it for patients, and discusses options and the benefits and drawbacks of various therapeutic approaches. In short, this professional takes responsibility for coordinating all aspects of the patient's care. It is this individual who presumably has the larger perspective, and who has insights into how the illness affects and will affect the child and the family. This professional is in an ideal position to develop an individualized management plan with the family.

The pediatric literature strongly suggests that the general pediatrician — rather than pediatric subspecialists or nonmedical service providers — is the appropriate person to coordinate the overall care of children with chronic illnesses. This same literature urges the general pediatrician to attend to the child's developmental and psychosocial problems. Despite such urging, very little time is actually devoted to these subjects either in medical education or in pediatric practice.

A number of very real disincentives keep many general pediatricians from providing what might be called an ombudsman service. Many chronically ill children have relatively rare problems that general pediatricians seldom see; thus these pediatricians do not feel comfortable in handling the medical aspects of such illnesses. In addition, it is no easy task to coordinate well child care, acute care, *and* care directed at an underlying problem. It is sometimes threatening to general pediatricians to communicate with subspecialists who are more knowledgeable about these particular problems than they are. It can be time-consuming and tedious to obtain reports from a multitude of other professionals and to guarantee that all recommendations for further evaluation and treatment are carried out.

In addition, it is also often costly for general pediatricians to care for chronically ill children. Pediatrics is a high-volume practice with low pay per patient visit. In fact, the average pediatrician in private practice sees a child for a well child visit every 10 minutes, and allots approximately five minutes for each acutely ill child seen. This is compounded by the fact that Medicaid and private insurance plans do not adequately reimburse general pediatricians for the time-consuming task of caring for chronically ill children. Although these financial disincentives are certainly not the only reason that few general pediatricians coordinate care for children with chronic illnesses, they are a reality and cannot be ignored.

Despite disagreement about who should fill the coordinator's role, there is consensus among professionals that one person must oversee all aspects of care. Children who receive the most fragmented and specialized services obviously have the greatest need for such coordination. Any person who has long-term involvement with the child and family may play this role quite effectively in my opinion. In fact, some communities have begun to train "parent professionals" (that is, parents of children with chronic illnesses) to coordinate care and advocate on behalf of other chronically ill children in the community. Another perspective is held by those who interpret Public Law 94-142 as a mandate for local school systems to assume the responsibility for coordination.

If general pediatricians are to be the professionals who provide coordination of care, incentives must be developed. During the education of medical students and pediatric residents, exposure to children with chronic illnesses as outpatients should be provided, and training programs that foster interdisciplinary collaboration and focus on the psychosocial aspects of illness should be developed. Training must also be directed toward helping the future practitioner to communicate effectively with parents and children, with mental health and social services workers, and with school personnel. Continuing education courses for practicing pediatricians should update them on new advances so that a sense of technical inadequacy does not discourage them from remaining intimately involved in the care of these children. In addition, reimbursement schemes need to be revised so that attention to psychosocial issues and coordinating functions do not result in financial burdens for service providers. Finally, in our attempt to streamline services and increase their efficiency, we must not forget the social origins of many devastating problems of children with chronic illnesses or our role in both perpetuating and alleviating many of them.

DISCUSSION

Lee Schorr: Dr. Weitzman has recommended that coordination of a child's care should be a general pediatrician. This conflicts with a plan tried at Fairfax Hospital in Virginia, where a team — either a pediatrician and nurse, or a psychiatrist and nurse — takes responsibility for communication about children's care because specialists have given conflicting messages to parents.

Evan Charney: I would like to make a mild defense of Dr. Weitzman's model because, even though it is imperfect, I still think it is worth very careful consideration. I would go so far as to say that if primary pediatricians or family doctors do not play the role of coordinator and communicator on behalf of chronically ill children, I really wonder what their role is or if there is a need in this country for primary health care providers at all. We are moving rapidly toward emergency room care or on-the-corner acute drop-in clinics, a trend which worries me.

What is in the favor of primary physicians? First of all, I think they can be powerful advocates in the medical system. Rightly or wrongly, there is nobody who can advocate with equal power to another physician, unless it is an organized group. In addition, I think primary physicians have the social contract, if you will, of seeing a patient over time, whether the patient is well or ill. And society has not given that contract yet to anybody else, including teachers or social workers. Primary physicians have gone through training, so they should know what the specialists are doing, and should not be overly impressed with subspecialists' technical skills. However, I see a lot of barriers to using primary physicians as case coordinators. For example, they are trained in a system which rarely lets them see a successful primary care advocate negotiate the system. Rather, they see the successful specialists handle the cases so that their natural inclination is to refer patients to the specialist.

Bob Chamberlin: As part of this model, is there back-up from the specialist to the general pediatrician? A lot of generalists' failures have been due to lack of adequate back-up when dealing with a rare condition. I think there is a lot to be said for this model because it transcends the hospital to the community, it transcends various technical needs as well as human and social needs.

THE PARENT'S PERCEPTION: ORIENTING PARENTS TO THEIR RESPONSIBILITY

Suzie Rimstidt

Yarrow, a mother writing for other parents about her hospitalized infant, said that doctors and nurses played an important role in her emotional roller coaster. She said, "A word from any medical personnel could send me soaring or crashing. . . ." I felt the same way six years ago when my developmentally disabled infant son, Phillip, spent more than four months in a children's hospital in Indiana. Some health professionals caused me to feel extreme frustration, loneliness, fear, and outright anger, but others provided me with comfort, support, respect, and education. I an neither yearning for a Dr. Welby-Dr. Gates, nor am I recommending a Kaiser computerized health plan for everyone. I do feel, however, that definite improvements should be made in sharing the responsibility for better child health care communications within our present system.

Procedure

Following Phillip's illness, I reviewed a broad range of medical and lay books and articles, and began writing about my personal experience in a booklet for parents entitled *Speak Up for Your Child's Health*. In this paper I would like to draw upon my experiences and those of other parents to present a parent's perspective in the following theses:

1. There should be mutual respect and participation between parents, children, and medical providers.
2. Physicians should save themselves time and communicate more effectively by utilizing educational materials and physician extenders.
3. Patients and their families need medical providers to recommit themselves to sensitive caring.

Finally, in preparation for this conference, I developed a parent attitudinal survey and distributed it to 35 of my friends. Although I cannot provide complete survey results here, quotations from those who responded will appear throughout my presentation.

Mutual Respect and Participation Between Parents, Children, and Medical Providers

George Bernard Shaw, in his *Doctor's Dilemma,* recommended that physicians be required by law to add, "Remember that I, too, am Mortal" to their brass plates. While a common consumer complaint is that doctors act like God, Vorhaus, a physician who writes about doctor-patient relationships, feels that patients are ambivalent in expecting doctors to be both equal and also supermen. Belsky investigated the medical mystique which some physicians assume. He feels it intimidates many patients and parents, and results in a consumer reluctance to ask questions or question physicians' decisions.

The women's movement, consumer groups, and the general human potential movement have made significant strides in encouraging self-reliance and activism, but I contend that the medical mystique is still very prevalent. For example, in my survey, I asked, "Have you asked all the questions you wanted to on visits to your child's doctor?" One nurse responded:

> No, the doctor seemed too busy — very rushed — also, I would have been afraid to ask questions for fear the doctor would think they were stupid. In the past, some doctors have made me feel my questions were rather stupid, and I am a nurse, so I don't think they really were.

One barrier to effective communication is medical jargon. Parents and children alike need explanations from medical providers in clear, understandable layman's terms. Medical jargon can be both frightening and intimidating, and it can even cause consumers to give up trying to significantly communicate with physicians.

In February of 1982, Rinzler reported on a consumer survey in which nearly half of those answering said that a doctor's single most important characteristic is taking the time to answer questions in understandable language. One technique physicians might use to help them eliminate jargon would be to tape some visits (with patients' permission, of course) and then play the tapes back to identify jargon. Another technique for which either physician or consumer could assume responsibility would be having the patient repeat the doctor's instructions in the patient's own words.

As I call for the development of mutual respect, I must emphasize my belief that parents must accept some of the responsibility for improving communications and for dispelling the medical mystique. One mother in my survey reinforced this contention:

> I feel parents must get over their feelings of insecurities and feelings that professionals are not to be questioned. You know more about your child in most cases than a person who's limited to seeing the child during short office visits, and so on. At least question your child's doctor and let him know you are doing so only because you want what's best for your child. I have seen mistakes happen in hospitals where parents were too reluctant to ask questions.

Another mother said, "Doctors aren't going to start volunteering information or speaking in layman's terms unless we as patients force this by being informed or at least asking questions and requiring second opinions."

Parents can and should learn to become questioners of medical providers. A simple but important prerequisite for the parent is to keep a small notebook and pencil always available to write down questions about a child's health as they come to mind. Levin even provides stock questions that can be adapted by parents who do not know what questions to ask.

If honest conversations between parents and physician don't resolve serious problems or dissatisfactions, the parents should seek another physician. This is important, because if parents and physicians are at odds, a child's illness may well be prolonged.

At the same time that the parents accept the responsibility of asking questions and insisting on answers in understandable terms, medical providers should give full consideration to parental instincts. A mother in my survey reported that after her daughter's surgery she never saw the surgeon until a later office visit; at that time, she was unable to convince him that serious problems remained. When these problems continued, this mother tried to reach the surgeon unsuccessfully for several months. She contacted three other physicians before finding a specific reason for the problems, which required another surgical procedure. Following this second surgery, her child began running a fever. One doctor told her, "Kiddies just run fevers sometimes after surgery." Not accepting this finding, the mother returned to her child's primary physician, who diagnosed and treated pneumonia.

Use of Educational Materials and Physician Extenders

Many parents would appreciate an occasional suggestion of where to read more about a medical or behavioral problem. I learned this when I found that I felt less anxious concerning the rare syndrome that had been diagnosed in our son after reading several articles about it. While preparing for this conference, I discovered *The People's Hospital Book* written by two physicians, Gots and Kaufman. Had it been published and available to me during Phillip's lifetime, the experience through which my husband and I passed would have been somewhat less perplexing. I stress the need for educational materials because the more knowledgeable the parents are, the more confidence they have to assume an active role in the physician-parent relationship.

Educational materials also have the advantage of saving professionals' time. Greenberg feels that physicians lack time for empathy, noting that the kind of "revolving-door" treatment provided by physicians who see from 20 to 30 patients in the course of an afternoon hardly allows for listening to what patients say or the meaning of what they are not saying.

But Jensen is not willing to accept the shortage as inevitable. He writes that the most insurmountable barrier to communication is the physician's attitude that taking the time to explore the emotional context of the patient's life is an unaffordable luxury. There is evidence to the contrary that doctors who practice this exploration of emotions do so with little or no increase in time and dollar costs needed for medical care. In fact, many researchers believe that quality time with a physician will produce fewer patient-initiated follow-up visits and telephone calls, saving the physician time in the long run.

Understandably many physicians, nurses, and social workers now feel overburdened with their patient loads and will legitimately question how and/or why they should add one more concern to their job description. Professionals may feel that healing — not education — should be their major concern, but the two are inextricable, and I do believe more education will mean less need for professional attention.

I also question why parents have to find a pamphlet dealing with the question of when to call a child's physician inserted in a woman's magazine in a grocery store; shouldn't all parents have written information that represents their physician's philosophy?

Paraprofessionals, physicians' assistants, nurse practitioners, nursing specialists, clinical specialists, and physician extenders are some of the labels given to those on a physician's staff who have specialized training to take over some of the physician's routine tasks. Use of such persons would help facilitate communications. In fact, a controlled study with one regular clinic and one that used a nurse practitioner found that the nurse-clinic patients showed fewer disabilities, fewer symptoms, fewer broken appointments, fewer criticisms of their care, and decreased use of other medical resources.

Another controlled study in a student health clinic evaluated what happened when a nurse's interview replaced or supplemented a physician's examination in an initial student-health evaluation. The study showed that students had a greater opportunity to discuss their problems, had a clearer idea of services available to them, and had a greater sense of the staff's interest in them as individuals.

Recommitment to Sensitive Caring

Criticisms of the dehumanization of doctor-patient relationships go back at least to the 1950s. A survey of business and community leaders about how well doctors met the emotionals needs of patients in 1951 brought some recurring criticisms, such as criticism of the assembly line approach, the need for better physician listening, and criticism of medical offices as being too impersonal. A college president from Indiana said, "In some areas overspecialization has put the personal relationships of doctor and patient on the same level as mechanic and automobile owner." A respondent on my survey said she wished her physician showed as much care and concern for her child as her veterinarian did for her dog.

I experienced this dehumanization personally when I inadvertently inconvenienced an intern. Due to a complex communication mix-up, I arrived at the hospital 24 hours later than expected with my two-week-old son. Since the staff pediatrician who had agreed to take Phillip as a patient was not in the hospital, one of the interns on rotation in the neonatal intensive care unit was assigned to admit our baby. While Phillip and I were waiting, this intern loudly complained to a nurse immediately outside our door about his unexpected and additional patient-intake assignment. He was also angry that I had brought no chart nor records with me. (My local pediatrician had personally met with the staff physician who was to be Phillip's primary care physician, and that staff physician had all of Phillip's records.)

After completing an examination, the intern emphasized again and again how extensive our baby's problems were. Although his assessment was accurate, his feedback to me seemed to reflect only his exasperation at having an increased workload.

How can impersonalization be changed to a more sensitive and caring approach by physicians, nurses, social workers, and others involved in children's health care? Apley's insistence that physicians accept the full responsibility for their interactions with patients and families has merit:

> Before the start of my outpatient clinics I say, and get the undergraduates to repeat out loud, "If any child cries it is my fault." They rarely do. If doctors in training have difficulty examining a child, they are asked to write, "I failed to obtain cooperation." Such breakdowns become very infrequent, if the doctors assume it's their responsibility to analyze and correct the situation.

The total commitment to caring implied in Apley's approach was what one respondent in my survey experienced as she recalled one of her best communications from medical providers:

> ... the tall, masculine doctor took my baby boy into his arms and held, cuddled, and talked to my baby; he admired my baby and his eyes glistened with pleasure as he checked him thoroughly. He gave me thoughtful counsel on what to be expecting in the next few weeks and strongly encouraged and praised the value of my breast-feeding. Most important of all he assured me with "eye-to-eye contact" that I was doing a fine job, and I needed that at the time.

Techniques to Improve Communications

To analyze their communication skills, medical providers might videotape some visits with patients. When informed consent is sought, such recordings are ethical and provide excellent teaching materials for students and experienced practitioners. In addition, feedback sessions might be a good idea for the physician who has enough self-confidence to welcome criticism. Furthermore, patient surveys or a suggestion box for patient use might be valuable tools for health professionals to use in evaluating communications if they are sincerely willing to grow and change when complaints are justified.

Some would ask, "Which would you rather have — warm, compassionate care to usher you into the next world, or cool, scientific care to pull you back into this one?" But this question evades the issue, for compassion and technical skill must complement each other if patient care is to be most effective.

As parents, we deserve more than the provision of technical skill. However, we as parents must also accept our responsibility in obtaining care for our own children's medical needs. We need to read, to learn to ask questions, to insist on understandable answers, and to consider changing physicians as a last resort when communication is inadequate. We must serve as advocates for our children despite our feelings of being intimidated, of being made to look foolish, or of being rushed and overwhelmed by other cares.

DISCUSSION

Andy Selig: Susie, I would like to reinforce one of the points you made. In my talks with families of handicapped children, it seems that what consistently emerges is mothers, fathers, grandparents, aunts, and uncles saying it would be helpful to them to talk to another parent or family that has been through something similar to what they are experiencing. When all is said and done, even well-intended professionals in many cases have not been able to help these families as much as other parents.

Evan Charney: I think we should talk about strategies to implement some of your ideas. In an institution where I work, I have not seen organized parents' groups going beyond their particular issue. For example, in our hospital, we have a group called Parents of Special Care Infants, and they visit all parents whose children are admitted to the intensive special care nursery. And I have wondered why we do not move further to allow parent advocates to talk to all parents of all children in the hosptial. Or even why we do not allow allied professionals to talk to all parents. In our hospital, for example, social workers cannot approach patients for discharged planning without the permission of the primary care physician. To me, that is absolutely irrational, but we as a group of physicians are too strong and parents have not pushed hard enough to change this rule. Since the source of power in an institution is the Board of Directors, which supposedly represents the community, I wonder whether some parents' groups have not moved to apply pressure at the hospital board level. I guess I wonder if the board isn't another site for advocacy by advocacy groups.

Suzie Rimstidt: I would think so, although in the past I have read that when parents have been put on advisory boards of clinics, hospitals, and institutions, it hasn't always worked too well. It did not work because the issues they were allowed to address were as insignificant as whether or not free toothpaste would be distributed.

Joy Penticuff: I recently read about a group of parents who did a survey in their community. They developed a list of the support services that they felt should be available in pediatric units, and then they sent a questionnaire to the pediatric nursing supervisor and also the hospital administrator asking whether these services were actually available. These were such things as 24-hour rooming-in, for example. Then they published their results in a local newspaper, ranking the hospitals they surveyed. The article said that this approach was very powerful, for it caused administrators to change policies very quickly.

Mary Ann Lewis: If current projections are right, in the future we are going to have many more physicians relative to the number of children. These physicians will be in competition for patients. So this may be the time when parents can really bring about change.

Bill Frankenburg: It is clear to me that if we want to make a change in the system to facilitate communication and thus to improve child health, we must do more than just change medical school or residency curricula. We also have to help parents see the role they can play. The thing that is not clear to me is how we can address ourselves to a mass program to change the behavior of parents in general, not just the parents of children with special needs. Do you have some thoughts about that?

Suzie Rimstidt: No, I do not have any easy, overall solution, but I think that developing parents' awareness is the first step.

Karen Fond: You suggested that perhaps physician extenders and nurse practitioners could be more helpful in the area of communication effectiveness. I was wondering why you thought nurses might be able to better facilitate communications than physicians. Is it because they seem less threatening and more approachable? Is it that they seem to have more time? Or is it that the majority of nurses are women, and mothers tend to be the primary caretakers of children?

Suzie Rimstidt: All the above, I think. I was speaking particularly to the point that physician extenders could provide some services, thus allowing the physician more time to provide other services.

PARENTS' GROUPS AND THEIR ROLE IN EFFECTIVE COMMUNICATION

Susan Kelley MacDonald, M.A.

Parents' groups representing a variety of children's disabilities have become fairly recent phenomenon in the United States. For example, in 1972 when Prescription Parents was formed, the American Cleft Palate Association recognized about 20 similar groups in the United States. Today, close to 100 cleft palate groups exist, and that number continues to increase.

Why? Parenting a child with a disability frequently requires very special sensitivities and knowledge, and can be a very lonely, confusing experience. Information developed for parents is often sparse and becomes rapidly out of date as medical advances continue. The medical community cannot meet all the needs of parents with a special needs child. Indeed, physicians and other specialists are frequently involved with their patients for a relatively brief period of time — usually during a hospital stay or brief clinic or office visit — while parenting is a 24-hour-a-day job.

When an infant is born with a problem, or when a child is stricken with a disease, most parents react with a mixture of anxiety, fear, sadness, confusion, and possibly even guilt. If the parents are to be effective in their new situation, these emotions require attention. One of the most important keys in attending to these feelings is effective communication between parents and the medical professionals responsible for the care of the child. It is on this premise that Prescription Parents was founded. I'd like to talk about this group today, because I believe it illustrates what parents' groups can do to facilitate communication and thus contribute positively to the health care of children with handicapping conditions.

Prescription Parents, now the largest parent group of its kind in the United States, was founded *jointly* by members of several cleft palate teams in Boston and a group of parents. The spirit of cooperation and open communication between professionals and parents with which the group began has helped ensure its success. In fact, today the group continues to be governed by a Board of Directors comprised of equal numbers of parents and professionals.

The four goals of the group are essentially communication-oriented. These are: (1) to be a "systems facilitator;" (2) to provide linkages (communication avenues); (3) to act as an advocate; and (4) to raise issues. Through a network of volunteers, Prescription Parents has been able to implement the tasks necessary to achieve these goals.

Parents' Groups as Systems Facilitators

A parents' group, such as Prescription Parents, can serve as an effective systems facilitator because of the diversity of problems which it confronts. The essential organizations (or systems) our group frequently brings together for common problem-solving are: various "competing" hospitals, innumerable social service agencies, insurance carriers, educational facilitators, and various government offices, to name just a few.

While these agencies may act in parallel fashion and simultaneously affect the life of a single patient or group of patients, they can be helped to converge very effectively through a parents' group such as ours. For example, when we first began our group, we discovered significant differences in the way that physicians, insurance companies, and parents defined "cosmetic surgery." We brought these groups together to agree upon a definition, an approach which could not have been as easily or effectively handled by a single parent or single doctor.

Another example involves our work with the various cleft palate teams in Boston who were having trouble communicating their recommendations for individual children to the local school system for implementation in the children's educational plans. The scope of this problem was too large and the time involved too great for individual physicians to educate each parent and/or each school administrator in which children with cleft palates resided. Prescription Parents established a program through which parents are referred to us; our representative works in cooperation with the cleft palate team with parents and the local school system to resolve communication problems. In addition, we have published materials which parents and teachers can share as a base for communication regarding cleft lip/cleft palate.

The Role of Parents' Groups in Facilitating Communication

Probably the most important goal of a parents' group is to provide effective linkages for its members. At least four areas where a parents' group facilitates communication come to mind: (1) a parents' group can help parents better understand their own emotions; (2) a parents' group can help parents better understand medical personnel and, conversely, can sensitize the medical community to parents' needs and concerns; (3) a parents' group can reinforce information provided by health providers, and can develop information written specifically for parents; and (4) a parents' group can bring parents together to share feelings, problems, and solutions with each other.

Many self-help groups have been founded to put parents in touch with their feelings by working with more experienced parents. As I have mentioned earlier, parents, when confronted with the trauma of the birth of a child with a defect or with the news of a disease contracted by a child, have feelings which cover a wide continuum. Some parents cope with feelings of grief, sadness, anxiety, confusion, and so on, very quickly; others need more time, while a few may never cope very well. It is in this area of coping that our group can report some success. Through our newborn program, an experienced parent (usually the mother) talks with new parents, and regular meetings of new parents are held under the direction of trained parents. It is at these meetings that parents are able to share problems and concerns, and ultimately gain a sense of competence and of coping. Parents report how much better they feel after talking and meeting with parents from Prescription Parents. They have reported relief at recognizing their own feelings in others, as well as seeing parents with children with problems similar to theirs who are coping well and whose children's habilitation is progressing.

This parent-to-parent contact not only helps parents cope with feelings, but also improves basic parenting skills which are frequently developed only through experience by parents of a handicapped child. For example, feeding an infant with a cleft lip/cleft palate can be a frustrating, time-consuming activity. New parents are frequently reassured when they share feeding experiences with other new parents as well as with experienced parents. Since feeding is the first and most basic parenting skill area, a new parent's perception of failure only makes adjustment to the birth defect more difficult. In addition, Prescription Parents publishes material on care and feeding for parents of infants with cleft lip/cleft palate to further reinforce what parents learn from group meetings and relationships with other parents.

A parents' group also helps improve communication between the medical community and parents in general, as well as in individual cases. In the broader sense, the regular meetings of the group, the relationship of parents and medical leaders on the group's Board of Directors, and the various programs in which parents and physicians cooperate all serve to sensitize both parents and professionals. In addition, members of various cleft palate teams address membership meetings regarding habilitation issues. These meetings not only reinforce information which parents may already have received from professionals, but also raise the parents' general level of sophistication about their child's condition. This improved understanding, in turn, contributes to more informed participation by parents in the care of their children.

Conversely, regular meetings between parents, the medical team, and the medical leaders in the field sensitize physicians to the problems routinely encountered by families. For example, I am very proud to be able to report that Prescription Parents has been active in bringing to the attention of the medical community the effect of hearing loss in cleft palate children on behavior, learning, and peer relationships. As a result of efforts such as this, physicians are helped to see the total child and the effects of a particular pathology on the child's daily life, an insight which can affect the kind of treatment prescribed in many cases.

One of the most important tools our parents' group uses to increase and improve communication is the distribution of written materials, many of which are developed by parents with guidance from our Medical Advisory Board. Publications for parents of newborns and older children tell parents of the various therapies and medical procedures which their child may need. These booklets — in combination with our meetings — reinforce information parents receive from physicians, and help parents frame their questions during consultations. The information also prepares parents for various procedures, particularly for their children's hospitalization.

Thus, through meetings, written materials, and parent-to-parent sharing, parents with a child with a handicapping condition are more comfortable dealing with professionals. The information they acquire tends to break down intimidating barriers to communication that parents often fear, and allows parents to assume a more participative role in the care of their child. Increasing the parents' level of participation frequently gives them increased self-confidence, which is communicated to the child. This whole process ultimately reduces children's fear because they see that their parents are in control and can help them understand what is happening, especially during hospitalization.

Probably the most vital communications function of a parents' group is establishing parent-to-parent contact. This includes contacts between parents with children of the same ages as well as parents of children of various ages. Most active members of our group agree that we have learned as much from each other as from medical authorities and books. Tips from an experienced parent on feeding a cleft lip/cleft palate infant are invaluable to new parents struggling with hour-long feedings; other parents' suggestions on handling cruel childhood teasing are invaluable; advice from adults born with cleft lip/cleft palate on their struggles as teen-agers are priceless to parents who are trying to understand their own children. Sharing information makes us better parents, helps us cope better with frustrating situations, and reduces the sense of loneliness that parents of special needs children frequently experience.

Parents' Groups as Advocates

A parents' group has yet another important function: serving as an advocate for parents and their children. In combination with strong support from the medical community, our group has accomplished much in the area of improved education, insurance coverage, and state programs. From our first meeting, parents identified problems with insurance coverage (particularly in the area of orthodontia) as a priority. As a group, and with strong support across many disciplines in medicine, we changed the regulations of Massachusetts Blue Cross/Blue Shield regarding extended benefits for the cleft palate patient, as well as regarding orthodontic services.

During the drafting of special education legislation, we strategically placed parents in leadership positions to assure that the needs of our children were not overlooked. We subsequently published materials for parents to use with their children's teachers and with special education administrators.

We also worked with the State Department of Public Health to improve state programs for children with cleft lip/cleft palate. Parents felt that some state programs were not accessible and provided care that was not coordinated. Since a child with cleft lip/cleft palate requires the services of many disciplines, the team approach is vital; but as our parents know, it requires careful coordination. Partly due to the urgings of our group, the Department of Public Health reviewed its entire program. Today that program is comparable to private care; in fact, it provides care regionally and by specialists in major teaching facilities.

These examples of advocacy illustrate the effectiveness of an active parents' group when there is a *cooperative* working relationship between the parents involved and the medical community. Many physicians treating our children applauded our efforts and provided effective testimony at the various hearings, but would have been labeled as "self-serving" if the parents' group had not been involved.

Parents' Groups as "Issue Raisers"

I have discussed how a parents' group can provide channels for two-way communication between parents, between parents and physicians, and with the larger medical and social services community. A more recent communications role assumed by Prescription Parents has been that of "issue raiser." Physicians and many medical specialists see that they may be unaware of the effects of a particular condition on the child's everyday environment. They may not be aware of the child's relationship with family, peers, teachers, and so on. Since our inception, Prescription Parents has brought many issues relating to children's lives to the attention of cleft palate specialists in Massachusetts, as well as to the attention of the American Cleft Palate Association, where parents have been invited to present such issues at national conferences.

Four particular examples come to mind: (1) Prescription Parents felt strongly about the importance of parents' groups and, through national exposure, was instrumental in helping to form groups elsewhere; (2) we have continually brought to the attention of medical and educational specialists the importance of the developing self-image in a young child and the role an integrated preschool plays in this development; (3) through documented observations by parents, we are bringing the behavioral dimension in hearing loss to the attention of cleft lip/cleft palate specialists; and (4) because of requests from parents and teen-agers, we are piloting a program to bring a discussion of teen issues to the young adult patient. Although similar efforts have been made by specialists and also by parents, it is clear from our discussions with adults born with cleft palate that this information is best received when written or presented by affected adults rather than by "outsiders." We are also developing tapes prepared by parents and former patients for teen-agers.

Although each of the roles of parents' groups which I have mentioned could be the subject of a separate paper, the point is that they are all efforts developed and directed by parents which substantially affect the treatment of children with cleft lip/cleft palate. The communication between parents, children, and treatment specialists which occurs in a parents' group results in the vital participation of *all* essential parties in a child's habilitation.

DISCUSSION

Andy Selig: I have often wondered how you organize self-help groups if the parents themselves do not have the initiative to get a group going or if the group is not formed around a particular diagnostic category or problem. Have you had any experience with self-help groups that have not been initiated by parents? For example, I have been involved in starting self-help groups where the initiation has come from a professional, but where we have been able to find parents with leadership and organizational ability to take it over.

Kelley MacDonald: Our parents' group began from the professional community. When our son was very young, his surgeon approached several parents who subsequently began Prescription Parents. But it was begun on very equal parent-professional footing, which I think is the most important aspect. I know several parents' groups which have failed because they did not have professional support; they came off as antagonists, and that is the kiss of death.

To answer the other half of your question, Joy mentioned a group of parents of children in hospitals that cover many disabilities. That group in Boston, known as the Association for Children in Hospitals, covers many, many disabilities. In fact, it even includes the parents of children who are going to be admitted for a tonsillectomy, and it has been very effective.

Unfortunately, I do not think groups are going to organize or exist very long unless there is a real motivator, like having a child with a cleft palate, a cardiac problem, or a congenital hip disorder. So I believe that groups like Prescription Parents and groups for hospitalized children should make a concentrated effort to reach out to local PTAs and similar organizations where there are large numbers of people. I say this because I do not think you are going to find lasting groups organized around the nebulous issue of advocating for well baby care and a child in general.

Evan Charney: I agree with you Kelley. We are very issue-oriented in this society, and your model is exactly the model the medical profession has used and been criticized for. It involves a group organized around a certain disease and a single issue, pushing the legislature and the insurance companies for special benefits. And it works; it works for doctors and it is working for parents. The challenge is how to translate that effectiveness into a broader kind of issue. There must be 10 parents' organizations in Baltimore, and if your child has one of the problems they address, it is fine. But if not, your child may "fall between the cracks." Are there parents' groups coming together to share advocacy or other skills that you know of?

Kelley MacDonald: In Massachusetts, an organization called the Federation for Children with Special Needs is an umbrella organization that addresses the child who has the disability that "falls between the cracks." But this group basically does not cover well child care.

Bill Frankenburg: Evan, there was an article in *Pediatric Nursing* by Lucy Osborn which told of a private practice in Utah in which they taught middle-class mothers. What they did, believe it or not, was to cut down on the time that the physician spent with the family doing well child health care. Then they would have a group session at which the physician or another professional from the office would answer questions and lead group discussions. So that is one model that has addressed well child health care. They tried the same thing in California with Spanish-American children from lower-income families, but it didn't work. They were not able to determine if it did not work because of the differences in ethnic groups or in social class.

Karen Fond: I was involved with that second group, and I think what happened was that the Spanish-American mothers really didn't buy into the group experience. They are very much more private in their sharing in health care settings, and they did not interact with each other. In groups, they all talked to the provider, but they did not talk much among themselves. In addition, we had a mixture of classes, and sometimes one of the experienced mothers would speak up in favor of breast feeding, and a new mother would take the comments as criticism rather than support. Also, it was a very transient population, and trying to get people to come together was difficult.

Lee Schorr: I am wondering about the composition of your group. Do you find that it is composed mainly of well-educated people? And do you find that you are able to affect what happens to less well-educated and lower socioeconomic families?

Kelley MacDonald: I guess in fairness I must say that we do not have a scientifically developed socioeconomic profile of our group. My opinion is that our leadership is certainly middle to upper middle class; it consists of people who have both time and commitment. However, in our newborn program, which was designed to attract new mothers, I can see a new group of parents who maybe are less educated and have fewer means, but who seem eager to assume a leadership role. I think that is healthy. But today our leadership is fairly traditional, as I think you will find is true with most parent groups, and I do not know how you avoid that.

COMMUNICATION ISSUES: THE CHILD WITH A DEVELOPMENTAL DISABILITY

Jean K. Elder, Ph.D.

We are here in order to improve communication among those who live with, advocate for, and treat children. Some of these children have a unique combination of complex, long-term service needs: they are children with "developmental disabilities."

My presentation will briefly explore the legislation which has shaped services for those with developmental disabilities. I will describe the evolution of the term "developmental disability," its current legal definition, and the difficulty in applying it to children. I will also discuss the role of the Administration on Developmental Disabilities in meeting the needs of children with developmental disabilities.

Evolution of the Term "Developmental Disability"

Although the term "developmental disability" is relatively new, it has undergone a number of changes in its legislated meaning over the past 12 years. Public outrage in the 1950s, 1960s, and 1970s at abuses in institutions served as an impetus for reform of the service system. In 1970, this social consciousness impelled Congress to enact the first developmental disabilities legislation.

The Developmental Disabilities Services and Facilities Construction Act of 1970 (Public Law 91-517) defined a developmental disability as "a disability which:

1. Is attributable to one of three categorical disorders: mental retardation, cerebral palsy, epilepsy, or neurological conditions closely related to mental retardation or which require treatment similar to that required for mentally retarded individuals;
2. Originates before age 18;
3. Is likely to continue indefinitely; and
4. Constitutes a substantial handicap to an individual."

In 1975, the Developmental Disabilities Assistance and Bill of

Rights Act of 1975 (Public Law 94-103) added autism to its list of categorical disabilities. It was not until the 1978 legislation (Developmental Disabilities Assistance and Bill of Rights Act of 1978, Public Law 95-602) that reference to the specific categorical disorders was eliminated and the functional limitations of those with developmental disabilities were fully recognized. Rather than respond with an ever-growing list of disabling diseases, Congress enacted a "functional definition" of developmental disability. The 1978 (and current) definition is "a severe, chronic disability of a person which:

1. Is attributable to a mental or physical impairment or combination of mental and physical impairments;
2. Is manifested before the person attains age 22;
3. Is likely to continue indefinitely;
4. Results in substantial functional limitations in three or more of the following areas of major life activity:
   a. Self-care
   b. Learning
   c. Receptive and expressive language
   d. Mobility
   e. Self-direction
   f. Capacity for independent living
   g. Economic self-sufficiency
5. Reflects the person's need for a combination and sequence of special, interdisciplinary, or generic care, treatment, or other services which are of lifelong or extended duration and are individually planned and coordinated."

This definition is similar to previous definitions in its recognition of the special impact of a severe, chronic, lifelong disability which has its onset during the developmental period (now defined as the period up to age 22 years). The new law altered previous definitions in three ways: it includes *any* mental or physical impairment; it lists seven major activities which are important aspects of functioning in "normal" society and which a developmentally delayed individual may have considerable difficulty in accomplishing; and it places greater emphasis on a developmentally delayed individual's need for individually planned and coordinated interdisciplinary services. With the present law, there are no specific conditions which automatically make a person developmentally disabled.

Since the change was made from a categorical to a functional definition of developmental disability, it has been found that the total number of people considered developmentally disabled has decreased significantly. The developmentally disabled population is more clearly defined as the most vulnerable and severely disabled group, representing approximately 2.8 million people (or about nine percent of the 39 million physically and mentally disabled people in the United States).

States and agencies have met with mixed success in applying this functional definition and implementing it in planning. The task is complex because service-providing agencies are more accustomed to providing services based on specific diagnoses. Quantified measures of these life skills have not been developed and consistently applied, even to adults.

Developmental Disabilities in Children

There are major problems in applying an adult-oriented functional definition to children. For example, it is very difficult to predict the eventual ability of a young child for self-care, self-direction, and independent living.

As we continue to apply the current definition of developmental disability to children, other problems are also apparent. First, the disability must be severe, chronic, and expected to persist indefinitely throughout the life of the child. This presents a particular problem in the case of infants and very young children. Except in unusual cases, there is an understandable and appropriate reluctance to "label" these young children and to predict the limitations or disabilities which they might experience throughout their lives.

Individual Planning and Case Management Services

A recent major development in programming for developmentally disabled children serves to facilitate communication between parents and professionals to maintain the parents' rights in decision-making. This is the legislated requirement of a written individual habilitation or education plan. This individual plan is a tool for improving communication between parents and professionals who are involved with a developmentally disabled child. It is also important that all persons providing services are aware of other services which are being provided concurrently. The individual plan includes goals (describing what the individual is expected to achieve); specific, short-term objectives; strategies for reaching the goals (these describe services to be provided and indicate who is responsible for implementing the plan); and evaluation procedures.

Each client, or his or her advocate or guardian, participates with professionals and service providers in habilitation planning. Since

1975, the increased use of individualized habilitation and education plans has resulted in greater sensitivity to individual needs and has improved communication among parents, clients, and professionals.

Another important aspect of services to developmentally disabled people is their need for a combination of special, interdisciplinary, and generic treatment. Developmentally disabled persons are likely to need many services throughout life. Because of their multiple impairments and the chronic nature of the disability, many individuals need the services of professionals and paraprofessionals from various disciplines working together, rather than independently, over a period of years. Effective communication among professionals is a necessary prerequisite for insuring that duplication is avoided and adequate services are delivered. Thus, individual planning and case management services are complementary aspects of the service delivery system.

The Administration on Developmental Disabilities

The Administration on Developmental Disabilities (ADD) is responsible for administering the Developmental Disabilities Act of 1978 (Public Law 95-602), which was amended by the Omnibus Budget Reconciliation Act of 1981 (Public Law 97-35). The mission of ADD is to assure the rights of developmentally disabled persons to receive needed services. Because this involves all services on a continuing basis, ADD and its state counterparts take the unusual approach of gearing their operation around existing organizations and services at the state and local levels.

The dollars expended by ADD are quite small when compared to the total of federal and state funds appropriated for the handicapped (Table 1). The dollar figures are relatively small in comparison because ADD is *not* directly program and service oriented. ADD has a mandate to oversee and monitor programs and develop and disseminate information. It seeks to help each state's Developmental Disabilities Planning Council monitor and coordinate services, and identify gaps in services which need to be addressed. The limited money available to each state is used to help fill gaps where services do not exist and to assist in planning for future needs.

In addition to the state Developmental Disabilities Planning Council grants, ADD also provides University Affiliated Facilities (UAFs) with partial support of interdisciplinary training programs for specialized personnel to serve developmentally disabled people. The UAFs also provide highly specialized diagnostic and treatment services which are not readily available in the community.

Table 1. State and Federal Funds

Appropriated for the Handicapped in Fiscal Year 1981
(Estimates in Billions)

Federal, Residential Services	$ 5.1
State, Residential Services	6.6
Residential Services Total:	$11.7
Intermediate Care Facilities for Mentally Retarded	$ 2.80
Supplemental Security Income/Social Security Disability Income	2.00
Other Medicaid/Medicare	1.70
Title XX	.80
Foster Care	.18
Public Health Service	.11
Developmental Disabilities	.06
Department of Health and Human Services Total:	$ 7.65
Special Education	$ 1.80
Vocational Rehabilitation	.15
Institutional Care	.90
Community Care	1.20

ADD provides funds to each state for operating a Protection and Advocacy System to protect and advocate for the legal and human rights of developmentally disabled people. In addition, special grants for Projects of National Significance (which demonstrate improved methods of providing services to the developmentally disabled population) are awarded each year.

In summary, the developmental disabilities program has, from its inception, filled an important role for disabled children and adults. Unlike most other programs, ADD's primary purpose is not the direct delivery of services. Rather, it is intended to serve as advocate and facilitator for planning, mobilizing, and coordinating existing resources so that they serve developmentally disabled people more appropriately, effectively, and efficiently.

The population served by ADD has always been that portion of the handicapped population which is least likely to receive adequate care from generic agencies or even from programs aimed specifically at handicapped individuals. ADD's efforts have brought together consumer groups, state agencies, and private nonprofit providers of services to provide a comprehensive network of services for the developmentally disabled population.

Inherent in this overall role is communication involving developmentally disabled persons, their families, and all others who have their interests at heart. The individual habilitation and education plans and case management systems have encouraged this process. Effective communication is essential if we are to serve developmentally disabled individuals well. That is ADD's mission. Clearly much progress has been made, but we have much yet to learn about how to accomplish our goals.

DISCUSSION

Bob Chamberlin: What can we and other professionals do to help get good legislation passed in 1984?

Jean Elder: The ADD authorizing legislation will come up for renewal in late 1984. Throughout the next 18 months there will be opportunity for input in this legislative process. In addition, there are other pieces of legislation concerning children which are currently in the 1983 renewal process; these include Child Abuse and Neglect Prevention and Treatment Act of 1974 and the Adoption Opportunities Program. The Head Start Act and the Runaway and Homeless Youth Act expire in 1984. As professionals and concerned citizens, you are encouraged to contribute your views on these and other pieces of legislation.

Bob Chamberlin: What is ADD doing about prevention? It seems to me that emphasis in this area is lacking.

Jean Elder: Prevention has been a focus in ADD since the original developmental disabilities legislation. At present many states have selected child development services as a priority area and have become involved in prevention activities. In addition, University Affiliated Facilities provide a variety of prevention services including genetic counseling, identification of high-risk infants and follow-up of development, infant stimulation programs, parent education, and training of professionals. Within the Department of Health and Human Services, the Public Health Service also provided an extensive array of prevention services.

Jon Ziarnik: I hate to sound like a broken record at this Round Table, but I believe in systems changes, and I believe that we need long-range planning for the developmentally disabled instead of the constantly fluctuating approach we have seen.

Jean Elder: I agree, and planning for the needs of people with developmental disabilities is a major role of each State Developmental Disabilities Council. Some states have been more successful than others at this. At the national level, our planning has not been as well coordinated and research-based as it should be. In ADD we are trying to overcome this by establishing a solid data base comprising population and service statistics which can be used to plan for developmentally disabled people in a more effective manner.

Lisbeth Schorr: We have the evidence that prenatal care really works in terms of prevention, yet prenatal care programs under Maternal and Child Health are being cut. And we have evidence that nutritional programs for pregnant women and young children also work, but these programs are also being slashed. It isn't that we do not have the data. We do have the data, and they show that these programs have been effective. So there must be some other elements operating here.

Jean Elder: There are a lot of elements involved. These are difficult economic times. We do not have unlimited resources in this country, and all programs face re-examination. With limited resources it is very difficult to establish priorities, and determine which programs reflect an appropriate federal role and provide the greatest benefit. These decisions are not easy, but they must be made.

COMMUNICATING WITH COMMUNITY-BASED CARE PROVIDERS

Jon Ziarnik, Ph.D.

As I entered the classroom, Pat Benson approached me: "When you have a chance, we need to talk about Billy's program." Pat was Billy's second grade teacher in a self-contained classroom for children with behavior disorders and I was helping her design a program to remediate Billy's behavior problems. As we talked, Pat explained that she had recently learned that Billy had been placed on "some medication to help with his behavior" by a pediatrician. She had noticed that Billy was acting unusually lethargic in school, and so had asked Billy's parents about the medication. They had been able to tell her little other than the name of the drug and of the physician. With the approval of Billy's parents, Pat contacted the physician, but her calls had not been returned.

A scenario like this has been repeated in virtually every community-based program with which I have had contact in the past 10 years, whether it be a regular school program, an infant stimulation program, or a program in a residential facility. The issue here is not whether a particular medical intervention was technically appropriate; rather, the issue is how the intervention occurred.

The service delivery system for handicapped persons has changed markedly in the past 10 years, a fact which physicians must recognize and adapt to. The purpose of this paper is to outline some of these changes and to suggest that physicians can work more effectively with education professionals.

This paper will not be a "how-to" communication document. There is a vast amount of literature on physician-patient communication as related to age, sex, type of disease, and race. In addition, there are numerous studies relating physician communication to treatment compliance and patient satisfaction. I have not made any systematic attempt to distill, categorize, or refine all these studies; nevertheless, I think we can safely conclude at this time that certain verbal and nonverbal communication skills have some relationship to certain types of treatment outcomes for certain types of patients. This is in no way an attempt to discredit the efforts of communication educators, but to point out that we are a long way from specifying — in any cookbook sense — *the* important communication variables. It is not a tautology to state that communication is a complex phenomenon. The complexity of interpersonal variables, including learning histories of the participants, make conclusions gained from studies at any one point in time tentative at best.

We do know that in order to adequately treat a majority of patients, a physician's technical skills alone are insufficient. For example, in 1972, Duff, Rowe, and Anderson found that only 12 percent of patients in a pediatric clinic were there for purely physical concerns, while nearly 36 percent were there for purely psychological concerns.

Furthermore, we know that in studies examining communication between physicians, parents, patients, and other professionals, almost everyone was shown to be dissatisfied — including the physicians. Beck and associates found that 40 percent of the teachers and 73 percent of the physicians were dissatisfied with the communication from each other in a school health program, while Ley found that 65 percent of the patients interviewed were dissatisfied with their physician's communication. Although it is easier to design research to measure "satisfaction" than to identify all the variables associated with it, one variable — "information given" — does seem to be important to patients. Physicians may be reassured to know that giving patients and others information has not resulted in an insatiable and unreasonable demand for information.

Changes in the Service Delivery System for the Handicapped

As I have stated, there has been a revolution in the service delivery system for handicapped children and adults in this country. What this specifically has to do with physician-patient communication is that the physician is no longer *the* caregiver for a handicapped child. Rather, the physician is now part of an entire team which is charged with the care of the handicapped person.

The 25 percent decrease in institutional population since 1970 has been accompanied by a rapid increase in community-based services. For example, a 1979 survey of 4,427 community-based residential facilities found that more than half had opened between 1973 and 1976. As a result, there are now many more children receiving specialized services from persons whose primary training and background is not health or medicine; instead, many handicapped children receive services from persons with undergraduate degrees in social work, educational rehabilitation, special education, or psychology. Furthermore, these persons usually are required by law, judicial mandate, or policy to be responsible for the direct delivery and/or purchase of specialized services. In short, a whole new system of community-based case management responsibility has recently evolved.

While many books and manuals have detailed these changes, we can summarize them as follows:

1. The first major change involves changes in teaching technology. Great strides have been made in the development of appropriate instructional techniques for severely and profoundly retarded individuals. We now know that systematic and data-oriented instructional techniques, based on learning principles, can enable handicapped individuals to acquire skills previously thought impossible. Our ability to teach these skills has resulted in the second major change.
2. The second major change involves increased integration of handicapped persons into existing regular programs (such as

programs in public schools). This has resulted in an increased need for liaison between professionals and regular school teachers and aides regarding the health needs of special children.
3. The third major change involves the development of specialized services in the least restrictive environment. Public Law 94-142, the Education for All Handicapped Children Act, and Public Law 94-103 (revised 95-602), the Developmental Disabilities Assistance and Bill of Rights Act, have provided much of the funding and mandates for the development of specialized services to handicapped persons. Thus, it is important for physicians to be knowledgeable about both laws.

Implications for the Physician

Given the recent and drastic changes in the scope and type of services available in the community for handicapped children and adults, there are at least three implications for the physician.

First, it is important for the physician to identify the ecosystem in which the patient functions. This ecosystem includes both the services (for example, school, residential, day care, or vocational training program) and the responsible personnel in each program (for example, school nurse, teacher, psychologist, physical or occupational therapist). Bryan and associates have identified six variables necessary for successful physician involvement in school programs.

1. The school staff must be knowledgeable.
2. The physician must provide the medical information school personnel need.
3. Each participant must respect the contributions of the others.
4. Time for communication must be available.
5. Predetermined forms and/or procedures which facilitate communication must be available.
6. Parents must be eager to help.

Second, the physician must identify his or her role in care of the handicapped child. As I have stated previously, some nonmedical groups have been made legally responsible for coordinating care for handicapped persons. As a result, Duke has suggested that physicians should adopt an interpretive services model. In this model, the physician usually acts as a consultant who integrates important medical information into all the services for a child.

Third, the physician (as well as others involved with the patient) must communicate for the interpretive medical services model to be effective. In a disturbing study, Cummins, Smith, and Inui found that physicians do not always even communicate with other physicians about patients. In a total of 233 referrals to specialists from a two-physician general practice, follow-up information was provided back to the referral source only 62 percent of the time. Even more important, follow-up information was received for only 54 percent of the patients where ongoing involvement by the referring physician was necessary. The study concluded by suggesting that "substantial improvement could take place if consulting physicians became more aware of the simple fact that the local physician is often a concerned, conscientious person deserving of better communication." The same could be said for teachers, social workers, psychologists, or paraprofessionals providing community-based care.

Beck et al. have suggested the following steps to better physician-educator communication:

1. Both parties must increase the exchange of information.
2. Both parties must clarify who will be the physician's contact person (for example, principal, teacher, or social worker).
3. Both parties must agree in advance on the information to be exchanged.
4. Both parties must specify a time to communicate.
5. The physician should attend school conferences which deal with medical concerns.

Communication is always subject to the variables brought to the process by the professionals, children, families, and other parties involved. Thus, it will frequently be imperfect. However, by understanding the changing face of community-based services, and anticipating the problems inherent in effective communication, we can move closer to ensuring greater continuity of care for handicapped children and adults.

DISCUSSION

Andy Selig: What can we do about the problem that results because a child may have five or six caregivers at one time, all giving conflicting advice, assessing the problem differently, and making different kinds of recommendations for treatment?

Jon Ziarnik: Public Law 94-142 went a long way toward an attempt to solve that problem by mandating that an interdisciplinary team with a case coordinator must decide goals and objectives for each handicapped child. Also, adult services generally have an interdisciplinary team and a case coordinator even though that is not a legal mandate. But what we need to do is somehow look at the economic structure that results in a disincentive for professionals in private practice to come to an interdisciplinary team meeting.

Andy Selig: Is there any way to ensure that the individual who takes responsibility for case coordination will be more educated? It seems to me that is important because not all professionals are going to be able to come to all the team meetings.

Jon Ziarnik: Well, most states do have somebody who is identified in the system as the client's case manager and who is charged with organizing information, but often that person has only a bachelor's level degree — sometimes less. Many of these people are in need of assertiveness training when dealing with professionals. It is very rare to find people with advanced degrees who are involved in community-based programs.

Lee Schorr: Is there any data that show that paying professionals to attend case conferences really helps? And, is that being done anywhere?

Jon Ziarnik: I am not aware that it has become policy anywhere, but I believe it would help. For example, my colleagues and I recently got a contract with one of the vocational programs in Colorado, and just the involvement of our group in this program has markedly changed the content of the case conference.

Kelley MacDonald: In Massachusetts, the law specifies third-party insurance payment for professionals like physicians to attend case conferences for children with special needs.

Bill Frankenburg: Sometimes physicians in private practice will charge patients for attending case conferences in schools. The problem as I see it is that you are dealing with two different worlds. Physicians often perceive that the schools have many professionals who have virtually unlimited time to sit around and talk. The physicians who are in private practice where time is money may attend a team meeting that may be long or not to the point. It can be a very exasperating experience for them. Another aspect that one needs to consider is that some problems are extremely simple and that it may not be worthwhile for the physician to attend team meetings. What we suggest to physicians at our Center is that they should decide whether the child's problem is simple or complex. If it is relatively simple, we say the physician could write a letter or make a phone call to school personnel; or the physician could communicate findings to the school nurse. In other words, we tell physicians that they must communicate with the school, but it may not be necessary for them to attend case conferences unless the child has complex problems.

Joy Penticuff: Perhaps technology can be used to get people together over distances. A simple thing like a conference call can solve a lot of problems, but we hardly ever use them, even though they are readily available.

Chuck Lewis: I would like to respond to that, Joy. A couple of years ago I took a sabbatical and went to the Andrews School of Communication at the University of Southern California in the hopes of finding marvelous devices that would improve communications in medicine. And what I found was that people who cannot talk to each other effectively face-to-face cannot communicate any better using technology. For example, at a video teleconference between California and New York, which costs about $1,000 a minute, somebody might say, "How is the weather in New York?" I think we have to be careful not to use technology as an escapist approach to effective communication.

WELL CHILD CARE

Robert W. Chamberlin, M.D., M.P.H.

One of the major goals of well child care has been the promotion of optimum growth and development. To achieve this goal, recommendations are usually made for periodic developmental assessments and for the provision of anticipatory guidance and counseling to reassure families and improve parenting skills. This paper will look at how well our current system of well child care carries out these objectives and the implications for the future. First, let us look at studies which have tried to determine the effects of guidance and counseling on parent functioning and on child health and development.

Studies of Guidance and Counseling

It has been reasonably well documented (by Casey and Whitt, Gutelius and associates, and my own work with Szumowski and

Zastowny) that mothers receiving care from physicians who provide more guidance and counseling learn more about child development, interact more positively with their child, and feel more supported by the physician in their parenting role than mothers whose physicians spend less time in these types of activities. Direct effects of these efforts on child health and developmental outcomes, however, are much harder to establish.

Part of the problem is that most physicians don't spend much time in guidance and counseling, as a number of studies from all over the country have established. The most extensive report was made by Rogers, who participated in a 1980 Quality Assurance Study for the American Academy of Pediatrics. In this study, a nationwide sample of pediatricians was interviewed, and well child chart audits were done for 150 practices. This study showed that the pediatricians placed counseling and supervision rather low in their priorities; in addition, by far the most common omission in the chart audit was the practice of health education and counseling. Interviews with the pediatricians after the audit indicated the omission of health education and counseling was an actual omission of practice and not just a failure in recording. A half-dozen less extensive studies involving office observations have documented this same finding. The latest of these involved a random sample of pediatricians in Pittsburg, in which the average time devoted to well child visits was about 10 minutes, and only 90 seconds of this time was focused on anticipatory guidance and counseling.

It would be easy to conclude from these studies that a major effort should be devoted to the training of primary care physicians in communication skills. However, this would not remedy the other major defect in the way we deliver well child care in this country, which is that the services often do not reach those families most in need.

Defects in the Child Care System

A number of studies, including one by Leopold, have shown that families living in environments characterized by high levels of stress and low levels of support are poor utilizers of preventive health services. That is, they do not come to physicians for well child visits. Most physicians are simply too busy caring for the families that do come into the office to worry about the ones that don't. Thus, pediatricians spend the majority of their time delivering preventive services to those families who need them the least. Even if some high-risk families manage to reach the physician's office, most primary care providers are not set up to handle complex life situations — and if they did spend the time necessary, it would be prohibitively expensive.

In this country, public health approaches to well child care also have major problems. While these providers are often more concerned than private practitioners about persons who do not reach pediatric offices for well child visits, their approach is often too fragmented by categorical funding to be effective. Nutrition programs are run separately from immunization programs, which are run separately from child abuse programs, and so on, so that it is impossible to approach the family in any kind of ecologically valid way. In addition, many public health programs are poorly coordinated with primary care, which is another complicating factor. Finally, public sector preventive programs have low priority for most communities, and are usually the first to be eliminated in a budget crunch (as is happening across the United States today). Therefore, if we are going to meet parental and child needs for guidance and support, I think we need to devote more time to changing the nature of the system as a whole, rather than concentrating solely on improving the communication skills of the provider.

An Ecological Approach to Child Health Care

I would first like to touch briefly on what I think needs to be done to improve the system. First, we must approach child health care from an ecologic perspective which recognizes that child health and developmental outcomes are related to parent functioning, which is influenced by both formal (health and human service providers) and informal (family and friends) community support systems. These formal and informal community support systems are, in turn, influenced by both cultural values and local and national governmental policies. Figure 1 illustrates this ecological model.

I believe that translating the ecological model into practical programs at a community level would require including at least the following five components (in addition to primary health care services): a needs assessment system, a community council, a health education program, basic parent support services, and a consumer advocacy organization.

A *needs assessment system* could be used to identify problem areas in the community and monitor program effects over time.

A *community council,* made up of representatives of consumers, health care and human services providers, community leaders, and government officials, could establish priorities and coordinate services.

A *health education program* could be designed to do a number of

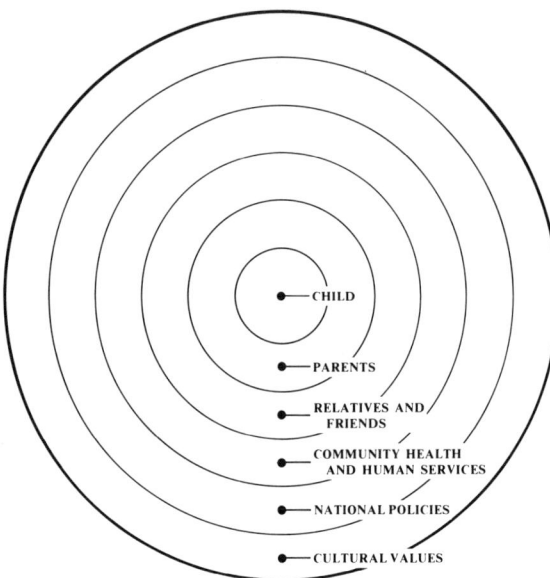

Figure 1. An ecological model of development.

Note—Reprinted with permission from "Prevention of Behavioral Problems in Young Children," *Pediatric Clinics of North America* 29(2):243, 1982.

things. First it could educate the community in general, and community leaders in particular, about the need for preventive/promotive services and their long-term cost-effectiveness. The program could also educate actual or expectant parents about what they can do to improve their chances for a healthy baby and to enhance the social and physical development of their child. And the program could educate future parents and health care consumers about what they can do to enhance their own health and development and that of their future children.

The availability of *basic parent support services* would encompass a number of diverse programs. For example, parent-child centers could provide parents with information about child-bearing and parenting, and could provide both quality day-care services during parents' working hours and temporary child care during times of stress. Birthing rooms or centers could provide an emotionally supportive atmosphere for parents-to-be and other family members during labor and delivery, and could help facilitate bonding through early and sustained parent-newborn contact. Home visitor efforts could help families faced with high levels of stress and low levels of support, since these factors interfere with a family's ability to make effective use of office- or clinic-based health programs. Homemaker services could provide emergency care when a mother becomes incapacitated during a crisis, and could provide home aides to help families over long periods of time when a parent or parents are unable to care for their children due to emotional or physical illness. And transportation could be provided to help families who live in isolated areas reach health support systems. This transportation should also be available when a crisis occurs and usual sources of transportation are unavailable.

A *consumer advocacy organization* could help monitor how well existing programs are meeting family needs. The organization could work with local government officials and others to insure the sustained long-term funding of service.

In contrast to Finland and Denmark, which have comprehensive community-wide approaches to prenatal and well child care, the best we have been able to do in this country (as Silver and Wynn and Wynn point out) is to develop comprehensive neighborhood projects that involve only a small geographic segment of a community, or a community-wide program that involves only a small segment of the total population (that is, those labeled "high risk"). Although both approaches have been shown to benefit those receiving the services, they do not cover enough of the total population to have much impact on the overall prevalence of various child health and development problems. We are, however, gaining some knowledge from these efforts which should help us develop more extensive programs when the need for them is more widely recognized.

For example, in one project with which I have been associated, a country-wide preventive/promotive home visitor program for young/single and/or poor mothers having their first baby has been initiated. We have learned from this effort how to successfully integrate such a program into the community network of health and human services providers through the formation of a community council and selection of nurse home visitors with extensive community ties. About two years of ground work was necessary to set up the coordinating mechanisms for the interprovider communication and cooperation that is necessary to get such a program off the ground. Now, as I have pointed out (with Olds and Dawson), almost every private practitioner and public agency is cooperating in terms of referrals and the coordination of services.

In summary, well child care in this country often falls short of its stated objectives. This is partly because many providers spend little actual time in guidance and counseling, and partly because the system fails to reach those families most in need. To remedy these situations, attention will have to be paid both to improving provider motivation and communication skills, and to changing the ways in which preventive services are delivered.

DISCUSSION

Mary Ann Lewis: Bob, child and youth projects are aimed at providing health care to the more disadvantaged people in our society. What kind of impact do you think those projects have or could have had?

Bob Chamberlin: Most of the projects that I have seen did not have an adequate data base and design for effective evaluations. While there is suggestive evidence in the literature that these projects have been related to a drop in infant mortality, true cause and effect relationships are very difficult to establish. When you are dealing with a whole system, it is difficult to separate a piece of it and determine what effect that piece is having.

Chuck Lewis: I am sure that many of us here today are enthusiastic researchers who count on obtaining evidence and data that will influence policy-making. But the National Academy of Science has recently released some studies of the impact of Great Society programs which I think are important to mention if we are talking about influencing policy. The Academy's publication was entitled *When Numbers Are Not Enough,* and it basically suggested that many things that we would like to prove are not provable given the structure of the real world and limits of research methodology in randomized control trials. On the other hand, we have too often turned up our noses at many qualitative evaluation techniques. These build a rich data base which is extremely effective in working with boards of trustees, parents' groups, and others. And I think the conflict between the quantitative and qualitative evaluation of researchers needs to be highlighted if this conference is to point at where one can influence policy, because my opinion is that there will never be enough documentation of how child health communications can be improved.

Bob Chamberlin: It is interesting to note that *most* European programs are not based on hard data concerning cost-effectiveness. On the contrary, most are based on perceived need by persons of influence.

Andy Selig: I would like to get back to the question of how to involve communities and give people meaningful participation in their own health care. This is particularly important to ensure the survival of programs once funding is gone. The public health literature is replete with examples of how programs have failed primarily because attention was not paid to the felt needs of health consumers. But it seems to me, and maybe I have picked up on your word or your phrase, that if we are trying to get people interested and get them to carry projects further, should we start with their felt needs instead of trying to get them to come our way?

Evan Charney: What Andy says — that communities ought to be organized around issues the people feel are important — makes classic sense, but I am not sure the success rates for those kind of programs is any greater. For example, health may be very low on a community's list of priorities unless everybody is dying in the streets of some kind of poisoning. People may tell you they have a higher priority for improving housing, food, and jobs, for example — and perhaps it is true that better health will follow.

Bob Pantell: A number of years ago I was involved with the Migrant Health Act, which clearly targeted health as its number one priority. But if you read closely the legislation's goals, you found that they had to do with widespread community programs. And very often the health aspects of the Act got lost in the "making-jobs" aspect. Another initial problem which was finally corrected was that the first community boards had to be reelected each year. Obviously, it is impossible to run a large, complex institution when the board turns over every year. So I think care must be taken in how legislation is drafted.

Kelley MacDonald: We have had some problems in our area which involve community boards as a rubber stamp to the professional community. If this happens, the project is doomed. We have lost several very good projects in Massachusetts because the boards were supposed to be rubber stamp boards, and one by one all the community leaders resigned because no one has time to waste. When legislation is drafted, the power that is given to community boards is crucial.

PART II
STRATEGIES FOR TEACHING BETTER COMMUNICATION

Papers presented during this portion of the Round Table dealt with ways that parents, children, and professionals can be taught to communicate more effectively.

Charles and Mary Ann Lewis first describe their efforts to improve the ability of children with asthma and their parents to communicate about the children's health. The program, which the two presenters developed, enhances communication by first giving parents and children common information, and then supplying a common set of symbols they can use to describe the causes of asthma attacks, the use of medication, and so on. A second project is a school curriculum for Mexican children living in the United States. The curriculum enhances communication by requiring the active involvement of parents, children, and teachers.

Another project is designed to help children communicate with health professionals. As it is described in Judith Igoe's paper, the program teaches children to be assertive health consumers and is most commonly presented by school nurses. Throughout her paper, Igoe refers to children as "health consumers" instead of "patients," stating her belief that health care visits must be joint problem-solving ventures involving professionals and families in a mutual participation model. This conclusion sparked debate among some participants, who feared that there are families for whom a mutual participation model may not be appropriate.

A somewhat different perspective comes from Earl Schaefer, who emphasizes the important role that parents play in child health and development. Professionals, he says, should promote child development by strengthening families' abilities to care for their children. According to Schaefer, health professionals may occasionally have to supplement a family's care for their child, but they should rarely supplant that care.

Two speakers — J. Larry Hornsby and Evan Charney — focus on training physicians to be more effective communicators. Hornsby believes that interpersonal communication skills training should be offered from the time future physicians enter medical school and throughout their training and practice years. He develops strategies to address when training should occur, who should conduct such training and how, and what the training should include.

Charney focuses on the training of residents. He feels that the stresses of residency and the developmental stages through which residents must pass make it essential that they be provided with support groups and with faculty members who will serve as sensitive and caring role models.

Susan M. Thornton, M.S.

ENHANCING COMMUNICATION AMONG CHILDREN AND ADULTS WHO CARE FOR THEM

Charles E. Lewis, M.D., Sc.D.
and Mary Ann Lewis, R.N., M.S.

The topic of this conference represents the intersect of two enormous domains — children's health care and communications. Our presentation represents a tiny atoll somewhere near the junction of these two great oceans of literature. We shall begin by providing some map coordinates or directions so that others may locate our position in this vast territory.

To pursue our geographical metaphor, Figure 1 presents a gross and oversimplified view of some of the areas within the Oceans of Literature of Child Health. Expressions of concern and exhortations for improved services constitute the Sea of Social Concern, the largest single mass of literature in both domains. It is separated from the body of social psychological literature by the Cape of Scientific Evidence. (Many well-intended task forces and advocates have foundered during a harsh and unrelenting passage around this Cape.)

Also within this Ocean, there is a large body of literature just off the Point of Professional Preparation. It describes the need for, and the methods of, improving the communication skills of health professionals. Occasionally this body of literature also examines the evidence of the impact of improving communications. Cost-Benefit Bay, a deep and natural harbor, lies between this professional prominence and Point Pragmatism.

We have labeled the growing body of literature representing quantitative and qualitative research on the working of health services the Sea of Health Services Research. Its exact boundaries are ill-defined, and many a well-intended young generalist has perished (rather than published) in its turbulent, interdisciplinary waters. It is limited on the South by the Cape of Disciplinary Obfuscation, which presents an enormous barrier to investigators crossing from one major domain to the other.

The Ocean of Communication Studies also consists of several discrete seas, each with its own unique ecology, reflecting a Darwinian pattern of evolution. The most important and relevant of these to the topic of this conference are the Sea of Social Psychology (already mentioned), the body of literature examining the communication process within small groups, and the Sea of Sociolinguistics (or that subset of studies of the structure and functions of language and the social variables affecting its use). Perhaps most familiar and relevant to this particular inter-ocean exploration, however, is the Sea of Developmental Psychology, the most scientifically explored and charted of all of the areas discussed thus far.

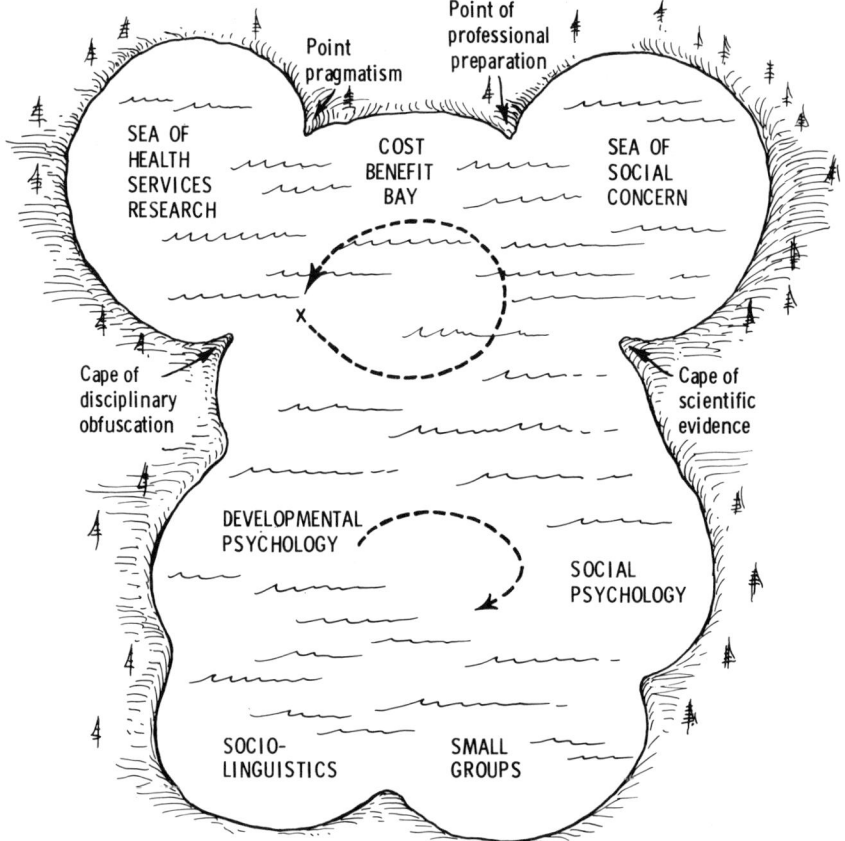

Figure 1. The Child Health Care and Communications Oceans of Literature.

As indicated on the map in Figure 1, there is a slow current or circulation in each of these oceans; we have suggested that these currents flow in opposite directions. As you will note, the tiny atoll (X marks the spot) representing our work lies somewhere in the eastern-most part of the Sea of Health Services Research, and closely borders the Ocean of Communication.

Research into Children's Health Behaviors

But enough of the metaphor. Next we would like to describe our research in a more traditional way. At the same time, we shall try to indicate the conceptual framework for the design of our efforts to enhance communications between children and their caretakers.

Our beginning efforts, in 1970, were concerned with the determinants of illness behavior in children. An inherent problem in examining children's illness behavior is that most of the interaction occurs between adults. Children are taken to physicians, who deal primarily with mothers (or other parents). The child remains passive in a process that requires active participation if a transfer of learning from one situation to another is to occur. These early studies focused on examining the patterns of behavior of children who were allowed to initiate their own visits to health care providers; we looked at the content of their communications with these providers, and their decision-making processes when they were provided with participating options (that is, "What do you think *you* ought to do?").

From this initial voyage into what remain relatively uncharted waters, we have mounted empirical and descriptive expenditionary studies. These explore certain questions related to the social context of childhood, and are by-products of our initial work. For example, what decisions do children believe they make and what things are decided for them? Are there any areas of joint decision-making in children's activities of daily living? We've also attempted to capture children's descriptions of the sources of distress that move them from the classroom to the school nurse's office; we have done this because in children, as in adults, psychological factors are the principal determinants of the amount of use of health services.

Our professional socialization and clinical orientations have led us to develop interventions whenever possible. Often these have been designed to treat symptoms rather than root causes. Like many of our colleagues, lacking insight into the actual causes of certain disorders, we have tended to provide well-intended, but semi-specific therapy. As a matter of fact, many interventions (not just ours) concerning communications with patients are somewhat reminiscent of the early treatment of syphilis (before penicillin). Patients were exorcised, over-heated, and/or poisoned in attempts to kill the spirochete/demon that afflicted them.

Our first intervention involved the development of a curriculum teaching elementary school children self-reliance and decision-making skills. We recently finished a national randomized control trial of this curriculum *(Actions for Health),* and the results will soon be published.

ACT for Kids

Over the past few years, our efforts have become more focused. We have attempted to combine the contributions of various domains of social science into programs that have rather specific goals. The first of these we shall describe is ACT for Kids, a program to foster self-management of their own disease by asthmatic children. The project, which was undertaken in 1979, was a collaborative effort between the Center for Health Services Research and the Center for Interdisciplinary Research in Immunologic Disease at UCLA. The latter group came to us because of our previous work in communicating with (or at least having listened to) a great number of children throughout the 1970s. The goal of ACT for Kids is to transfer the responsibility for the management of the child's asthma from parent to child; the objectives of the program are to reduce unnecessary use of emergency rooms, to reduce unscheduled visits to physicians, and to produce an overall reduction in the level of disability of the children.

This intervention was based upon improving communication, not just because it was a good idea, but with an eye toward achieving certain aims. We knew that if we were to achieve our objectives, we would have to lower both children's and parents' levels of anxiety associated with asthmatic episodes, and that we would have to increase their belief in the efficacy of their treatment and their belief in their own ability to prevent or limit the severity of episodes. We recognized that both parents and children needed a certain amount of information so that they would understand the aggravating factors which set off asthmatic episodes. We also knew that effective treatment required some degree of understanding and insight by the family into the meaning of the disease to the patient and the family. (For example, do the episodes constitute an excuse for the child to assume a sick role or a chance for adult family members to encourage learned helplessness, or are the episodes so threatening to "normality" that they tend to be denied?)

We were aware of the literature which suggests that simplification of information by practitioners for patients enhances the quality of communication and the potential for changes in behavior. Furthermore, we were aware of literature which indicates that teaching strategies for cognitive control (that is, self-talk, or mental exercises one can do when faced with symptoms) is important to enhance a patient's sense of control. In addition, the literature indicated that behavioral control strategies, such as relaxation exercises, should help promote that sense of control. There also were structural constraints with which the program had to deal, such as insuring that children have access to their drugs. Finally, we taught some decision-making strategies — not just because they're a favorite of ours — but also because we felt that too often families faced with the problem of having a cat and a child who was allergic to that cat thought of only two options — either getting rid of the child or the cat. In fact, there are several other alternatives. Once patients go through a decision balance sheet, they often decide upon more moderate arrangements than otherwise might have resulted.

In choosing to work with both children and parents, we were dealing with two separate groups of participants in differential stages of language acquisition and cognitive development. Therefore, the lesson plans (with the same content) had to be taught separately to children and adults. Because studies by Hovland and Weiss demonstrated the importance of the perceived credibility/trustworthiness of the message source, we agreed that physicians had to be involved, at least nominally, in these sessions. This agreement was reached although our experience has been that physicians are usually poor teachers; they know too much, and tend to give grand-round lectures in response to simple questions. We therefore reached a compromise: the doctor is involved only in the third of five sessions. In this class, each child's medications are individually reviewed with children and their parents in terms of dose, indications, and side-effects. With this exception, the classes are taught by a nurse clinician with a background in respiratory disease, who works with the parents, and a primary school educator-teacher, who runs the children's group.

One of the goals of the parents' groups is a shift in norms, to legitimize giving children access to their own medication. This change is much easier to bring about when discussion is by a group of five to 10 parents, one of whom has already allowed their child to control the drugs and can thus testify to the potential benefits and lack of risk of this approach.

The key to the success of ACT for Kids, however, is the use of a simple paradigm that facilitates communication through simplification. We chose the subtitle, "You're in the Driver's Seat," because the lessons are built around the concept of driving safely and recognizing traffic signals. Specifically, red means "stop," yellow means "slow down" or "watch out," and green is for "go." Children learn to identify their aggravators or sources of allergens by fixing green, yellow, and red stickers on various drawings, such as those shown in Figure 2. For some children, the dog may be a "red" aggravator, while for others the dog poses little or no problem, so it's a "green."

This strategy also permits an enormous simplification in classifying the medications used in the treatment of asthma. Some are prophylactic; that is, they are used to prevent bronchospasm when exercise is

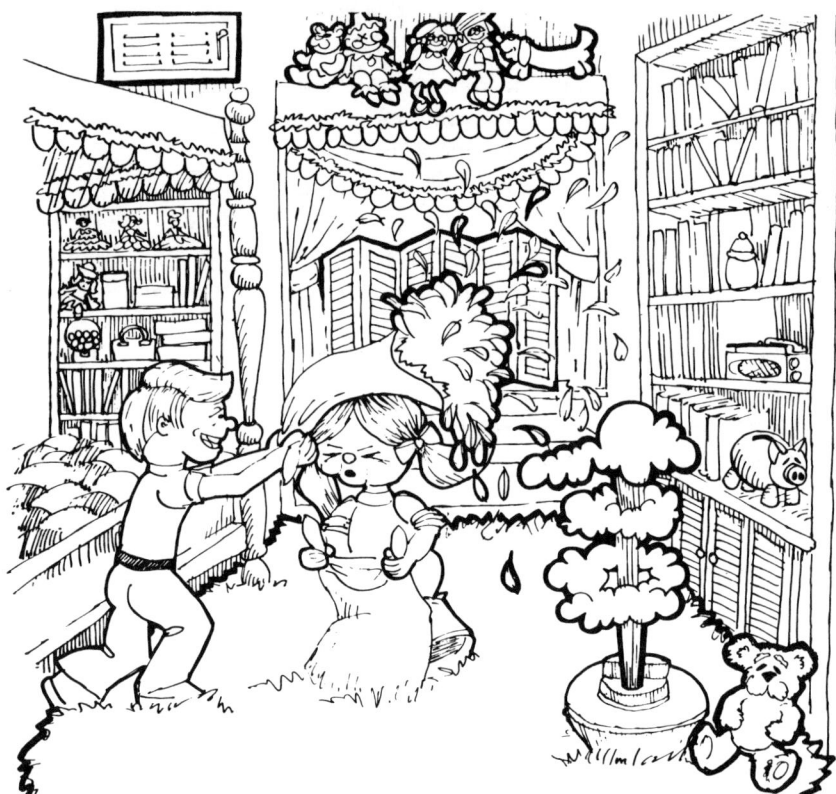

Figure 2. The Search for Environmental Aggravators (from ACT for Kids).

planned, so these are "green" medicines. The "red" medicines are used to stop an attack, or when there are severe symptoms.

We are just completing a randomized clinical trial of this curriculum at Kaiser Permanente in Los Angeles with approximately 45 patients in each of the control and treatment groups. The evidence thus far suggests that there is a significant reduction in emergency room visits and a reduction in the sense of panic associated with episodes in the experimental group. We are comparing the experimental group to a group which received a three-hour didactic lecture by an allergist. The lecture covered the same content, but packaged the messages in a different way.

Perhaps the most interesting outcome of the study has been the spontaneous report by families in the experimental group of increased communication between parents and children. They say they communicate better not only about asthma, but also about many other issues in their lives. It seems that having given parents and children a rather simplistic set of symbols with which to communicate about their disease has helped reduce barriers to adult-child communication in other areas. (Perhaps it has simply served to stimulate such communication in the absence of any "barriers.")

While we are just completing the evaluation of the "ACT for Kids" program's ability to improve communication within families of asthmatic children, we are near the mid-point in another study. We shall briefly mention this second study, because it also uses a specific strategy to improve communication between certain groups.

Circle of Care

In 1980, we began work under the sponsorship of the Rosenberg Foundation of a curriculum which we've called Circle of Care — I Care for My Family, and My Family Care for Me. It was intended to be a curriculum supplement for schools near the southern American border that serve children from Mexican families. Our initial expectation was that in many of these families, during times when both parents were working, children might be forced into assuming such adult roles as child care. We thus started out to develop an American version of the Child-to-Child program of Morely, which has been described by Aarons and Hawes. Morley's program has spread throughout the developing countries of the world, and is based on the assumption that the only individual who can be counted on to take care of an infant is an older child. Therefore, children are taught skills related to nutritional assessment, rehydration of infants with diarrhea, and so on.

As we edged into the Circle of Care project, we recognized that we had not defined a specific set of objectives, as we had done in the asthma program. In addition, we did not have a real feeling for the nature of the "problems" that we were addressing. Thus, we chose to develop a "safe" set of lessons for the first year that dealt with safety and first aid. We also wrote a unit we called "El Arbor de los Zapatos" (The Tree of Shoes), which was designed to help children identify the multiple role functions that family members play. However, we were concerned because we lacked information about who did what with reference to household duties in these families. We managed to find two graduate students in anthropology, moved them to San Ysidro, California, for the year, and conducted an ethnographic study of families of first, third, and sixth grade children.

From this we learned that the pattern of communication between school and families was very dysfunctional. For example, as shown in Figure 3, teachers communicated with children as best they could (these were bilingual classes), and they occasionally communicated with parents, usually at times when there were problems. Parents generally responded to problems by going directly to the head of the

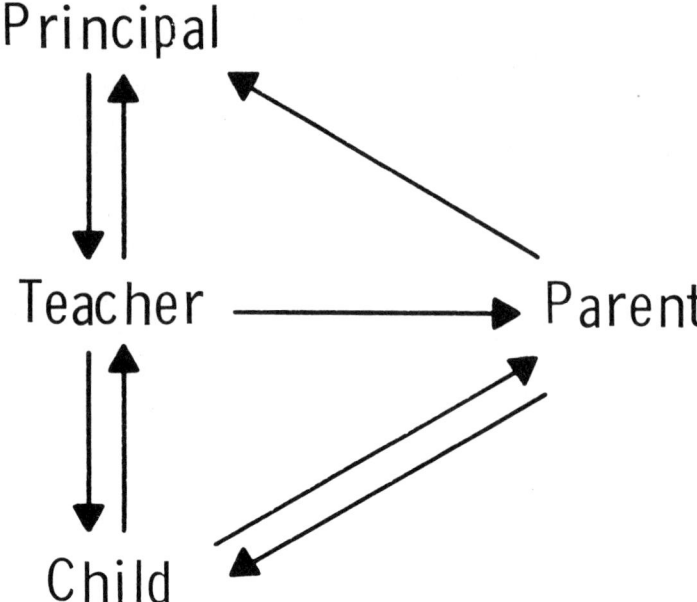

Figure 3. Dysfunctional Communication Pattern.

organization, the principal, rather than to the teacher. Presumably there was a fair amount of communication between the principal and the teachers.

One of our Circle of Care lessons, preparing a family tree, required children to do homework *with* their parents. This proved to be enormously popular both with the children and parents. Subsequently, it finally occurred to us that the goal of the curriculum we were developing should be to enhance communication between parents *and* children *and* teachers. This was done by designing certain lessons requiring homework, where the only "right" answers could come from the parents, be reported back through the children to the teachers, and shared with the entire class. Clearly, one objective of this study is to alter the existing pattern of communication to that illustrated in Figure 4.

The ethnographic studies revealed that while this strategy excited parents and children, it presented a problem for some of the teachers. This should not be surprising when one realizes that the information being brought back about the cultural heritage of these children may be in direct conflict with some teachers' previously held opinions (or biases). The result is what has been labeled "cognitive dissonance."

The Circle of Care curriculum to be field tested this fall will involve two experimental schools and a third school as a control. It has four major units: family roles, food and nutrition, games and recreation, and safety and health. In each of these modules, there are lessons

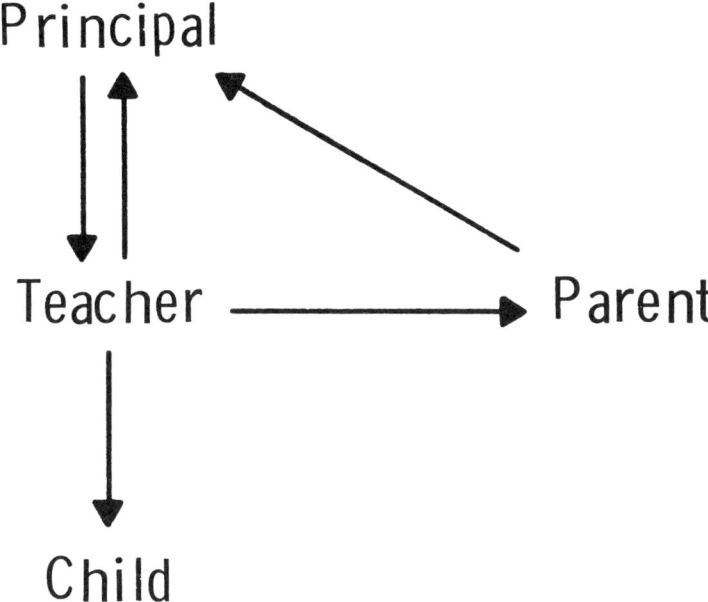

Figure 4. Desired Communication Pattern.

requiring that homework be done jointly by parents and children. For example, the parents must provide information on members of the linear family and their birth places, and on the family's favorite recipe, including family recipes (rules) for living. Other lessons explore the family's favorite games (played by parents and grandparents when they were children), and the safety mapping of households by children and parents who review drawings such as that illustrated in Figure 5. Together they identify and correct hazards that might be present for younger family members.

The public schools represent the promise of a better future for new citizens of the United States. They are also a major source of social stress, particularly as children are rapidly acculturated and move away from their parents' values. By providing children of Mexican families living in the United States with information about the strengths and values of their native heritage, we hope to increase the children's sense of identity. At the same time, we'll settle for communicating about safety, first aid, nutrition, and a few other topic areas yet to come.

Balancing Communication Research and Common Sense

In summary, we would like to suggest that attempts at improving or enhancing communication between children and the adults who care for them should be based upon clear definitions of the desired

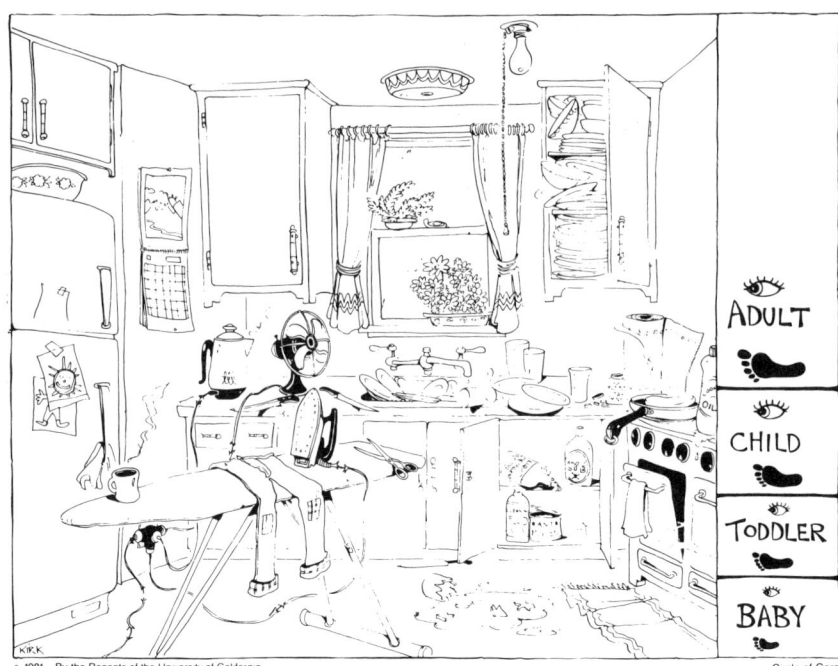

Figure 5. Safety Map from Circle of Care.

outcomes. In addition, both the design of such communications and the messages should be based upon the bodies of literature that exist in the vast territory we have described.

In "Talking to Children — Language Input and Acquisition," Brown of Harvard provides some scientifically sound advice. He answers the question of how a concerned mother can facilitate her child's learning of language as follows:

> Believe that your child can understand more than she or he could say, and seek above all to communicate. To understand and be understood, to keep your minds fixed on the same target. In doing that without thinking about it, you will make 100 alterations in your speech or actions. Do not try to practice them, as such, because there is no set of rules of how to talk to a child that can even approach what you unconsciously know. If you concentrate on communicating, everything will follow.

Perhaps health professionals focus *too* much on how to alter their speech to communicate with children, rather than relying upon their native insights. We do not know of any studies that compare how physicians or nurses speak to patients versus how they speak to their own children, but we suspect there are profound differences. Much of what we may hope to achieve in the future in this area may be a cross between doing what comes naturally, and doing it within the structure of strategies based on scientific evidence.

DISCUSSION

Barbara Korsch: I am very impressed with your presentation and just wonder whether decreasing the anxiety levels of children with asthma and their families is completely positive. For example, some might argue that a certain amount of anxiety is needed if the child is to get health care.

Mary Ann Lewis: Children tell us that at the onset of an episode of wheezing, they become so fearful that the entire family becomes fearful, and everyone gets very agitated. So what we have done is to develop a communication format which helps children understand and listen to their own bodies and know what is happening at the time, or just before wheezing episodes occur. We have developed "body maps" which help children learn that some children have tickles in their ears before an attack of wheezing, some have tickles in their throats, and so on; there are many such symptoms that I as a health professional never really knew until I heard children talk about them. When the child has identified that an attack is imminent, the goal then is for the child to take certain medication.

Barbara Korsch: You also stated that parents and children are equal now in terms of their understanding of asthma, and I just want to raise a theoretical question: Is that necessarily a desirable goal? At what point does the child feel less cared for by those who should, after all, be seen as caretaker?

Mary Ann Lewis: I guess what we have tried to achieve is some balance in terms of who is in control at what point in time to deal with asthmatic episodes. In general, parents have more information than children, which creates an unequal situation in which parents tell children what to do. This is not the best way for children to learn, for we know from learning theory that children learn best when they discover on their own. In addition, inequity between what parents and children with asthma know can lead to over-dependency and other maladaptive relationships.

Bob Pantell: I am curious, first of all, about whether you have qualitative information about the effectiveness of ACT for Kids, such as improvement in school attendance. Secondly, since your outcome measures really have to do with children interacting with the medical system, did you get any reports about what was going on in the physician's office?

Mary Ann Lewis: Number one, the criteria for selecting the children in our trial was that they be on medications at least 25 percent of the time. So it was a fairly sick group of children, many of whom missed a lot of school. When an asthmatic child gets sick at school, the first thing the teacher does is send the child to the principal's office because there is no school nurse most of the time. The principal's secretary then sends the child home. Yes, we know there was a qualitative change, because families tell us that their children are going to school and staying there.

Chuck Lewis: We have some incredible stories of children who have "taken charge" of their own lives. These are children whose pulmonary function studies have become normal, whose medications have been reduced, and who have gained weight. Some of the stories are almost unbelievable, in fact. The only reason we believe them is that all of the children were part of a Kaiser plan, which makes it easy to look up their medical records. This means we do not have to depend just on self-reporting.

Mary Ann Lewis: We conducted the pilot for this project in a group of private immunologists' office. What we found was that after the pilot, children began calling the pediatric allergists on their own, directly from school and from home. They began talking to the doctors, saying, "Look, this medicine is not working for me anymore." And the physician would say, "Okay, we'll switch. I'll order the prescription, and your parents can pick it up." Doctors have told us that the impact in many children was really fantastic, and *whatever* we did, it worked.

Lee Schorr: Would you talk about the difference in work you have done where you have been able to structure parent participation, as you have in the ACT program, and some of your other work at school with a more general population which did not involve the parents as intensely or at all? It seems to me that when parents are made partners in a program, it is much easier for them to think about giving the child more control over an illness, over relationships with the doctor, and so on.

Mary Ann Lewis: We have involved parents in a number of our programs, but it is difficult to try to involve parents in the schools. We think it is important to involve them, but it is very hard.

Chuck Lewis: We have found that we are able to change children's beliefs and their understanding and knowledge significantly, but we do not see behavior change until we bring their parents into the program. So you raise an important point.

TRAINING NURSES

Judith Bellaire Igoe, R.N., M.S.

Editors' note: Because Judith Igoe was unable to be present, her paper was read by Joy Penticuff, R.N., Ph.D.

Establishing a helping relationship is basic to all nursing care, and reflects the nurse's ability to assist parent and child in coping with stressful health-related situations. At the same time, the end product of such relationships should be the family's acquisition of knowledge, confidence, and self-awareness so that they are capable of greater self-direction in caring for their future needs. Wold has observed that it is possible to provide an atmosphere in which this kind of learning can take place only when appropriate communication skills are utilized.

While communication skills are complex behaviors influenced by such factors as attitude, experience, and personality, it is generally assumed by nurse educators that knowledge and understanding of the communication process can contribute significantly to the nurse's effectiveness in helping relationships. For this reason, past and current teaching in nursing is heavily laden with communication courses. Variables involved in communication such as perception, feelings, language arrangement, facial expressions, gestures, attention, comprehension, and nonverbal feedback are closely examined, as are other communication characteristics. In most instances, the instructor makes use of a variety of teaching strategies besides the customary lecture method. For example, films are often used to show desired communication skills, with students subsequently imitating the observed behaviors in simulated situations. Role playing is another common teaching method for improving communication, as is the use of audiotapes and videotapes so that students can immediately review and critique their communication skills.

Unfortunately, there is a disturbing issue that arises in many of these research studies dealing with nurses' communication skills. The research fails to indicate that nurses in general are utilizing the kind of communication skills in their work with families which would foster development of the family's independence and the use of their own support systems. For example, Kalisch has expressed concern that nurses often — both verbally and nonverbally — control adults and cast them into childlike roles. Nursing educators may find some consolation in the findings of similar studies involving other health professionals, which reveal the same tendency to encourage dependency. However, the long-standing belief of nurses that one of their special contributions to the field of health is in helping people to help themselves makes it impossible to disregard this practice flaw simply because other professionals are experiencing similar difficulties. New approaches to improving nurses' ability to establish more effective and reciprocal relationships with families are clearly needed.

An Experimental Approach to Teaching Communications to School Nurses

The University of Colorado School of Nursing's School Health Programs has spent the last several years experimenting with a different approach to teaching communication skills to experienced school nurses. Faculty members reasoned that, if the desired outcome was the development of relationships in which families and their children felt a greater sense of responsibility for themselves, then one of the key factors in achieving that goal had to be to increase their participation in the relationship with the nurse. Several attempts to get this concept across by incorporating it into the customary study of the process of communication proved to be largely unsuccessful. Possibly this was because the nurses involved were already familiar with the basic principles of communication and tended to consider this course content as little more than review. Under these circumstances, their style of relating to families remained essentially unchanged. Consequently, the decision was made to reorganize course content and begin from an entirely different perspective.

This time, faculty began by introducing Szasz and Hollender's conceptual framework (Table 1) depicting typical roles and relationships which emerge when health providers and consumers encounter one another in clinical settings. Within this framework, four areas suitable for further study became apparent. These were:

1. What is the goal of a visit for professional health services?
2. Under what circumstances is it appropriate to use a particular role/relationship model?
3. Given the goal of a visit for professional health care, are the

most appropriate role/relationship models actually in use in health settings?
4. Given the basic principles of communication, what are the similarities and differences in the ways these skills are used when different models of roles/relationships are operating?

Table 1. Roles/Relationships of Health Consumers/Providers

Model	M.D./ R.N./ D.D.S. Role	Health Consumer Role	Clinical Application of Model	Prototype of Model
1. Active-Passive	Do Something to Consumer	Recipient (unable to respond or inert)	Anesthesia, Acute Trauma, Coma, Delirium	Parent/ Infant
2. Guidance-Cooperation	Tell Consumer What to Do	Cooperator (obeys)	Acute Infectious Processes, etc.	Parent/ Child
3. Mutual Participation	Help Consumer to Help Himself	Participant in "Partnership" (uses expert help)	Illness, Injury Preventive Health Care Chronic Health Conditions Psychological Care	Adult/ Adult

Note—Reprinted with permission of the *Archives of Internal Medicine* 97:586, 1956, copyright 1956, American Medical Association.

When the instructional content about communication was placed within the context of health provider/consumer relationships, the nurses reported that the material was far more relevant to their practices. Follow-up observations suggest that, indeed, nurses are now enabling families (including children and youth) to become more involved and increasingly independent than had been previously reported. Altering the nursing training has apparently made some difference in communications patterns and for this reason, the training program merits additional description.

Barriers to Implementing Positive Communication Models

I have stated that nurses need to foster greater self-reliance and independence among the people with whom they work, and that certain communication patterns might be barriers to realization of this goal. This is true despite the fact that a review of the communication theories and models taught in nursing schools throughout the country indicates that course content per se is accurate and current. In addition, there is general agreement among nurse educators regarding the ways to improve effective communication. Evaluation of the students' knowledge of communication processes and the basic principles involved shows that the nursing students understand the information, and are far more proficient than nursing students in prior times. Why, then, don't they apply this knowledge in their practices?

A number of factors are involved in this lack of application and I will explore these soon. First, however, it is important to point out that the nurses' difficulty in communicating does not appear to permeate all three models described by Szasz and Hollender. Indeed, the major difficulty seems to involve the nurse knowing how and when to move the relationship from a guidance-cooperation model to the mutual participation prototype. This occurs despite the fact that classroom course content has emphasized the importance of guiding relationships with patients in this direction.

Some of the factors which the School Health faculty at the University of Colorado suspect contribute to this frustrating situation include the following:

1. There is failure to clearly teach student nurses that a visit for health services should be a problem-solving venture for the health consumer as well as the health professional.
2. The health care delivery system does not reinforce participatory relationships between professionals and consumers.
3. Communication between members of the health care team has often not been free and open.

The first point has been that there is a failure to clearly teach nursing students that a visit for professional health services should be as much a problem-solving venture for the health consumer as it is for the professional. Those who teach future nurses must be prepared to justify the need for this approach, and students need time to discuss, digest, and reflect fully on its implications.

There are a number of rationales, which nursing instructors must be prepared to present, for this approach. First, the nature of today's health problems simply cannot be cured by a single visit to a health facility. In most instances, consumers have to be committed to carry out their own health plans on a daily basis. Unless consumers have had some first-hand involvement in the formation of these plans, they will have no sense of ownership in them and will be unlikely to follow professionals' recommendations. To avoid noncompliance, health professionals and consumers have to work together to define the problem, to generate various approaches to solving it, to establish criteria for selecting the best alternative, and to design a specific treatment plan as well as a method for evaluating the plan's effectiveness.

The second rationale for encouraging mutual consumer-professional participation concerns the compliance failure professionals have experienced from merely doing things to patients or telling them what to do. The outcomes from relationships where both parties continually participate tend to be far more positive.

I should note here that it is much easier to explain mutual participation models than it is to put them into action. In some areas of the country, we still unfortunately tend to socialize students into their professional role as nurses with the understanding that they must always be in control. On the other hand, the average health consumer is ill-prepared to settle comfortably into the mutual participation model without a great deal of encouragement, instruction and support. (One possible way to combat the problem of neither consumers nor providers being familiar with mutual participation would be to train the two groups together in communication courses.)

The second barrier to participatory communication is that the present health care delivery system is not organized to positively reinforce participatory relationships between health providers and consumers. As a result, attempts to encourage these new behaviors are usually isolated and involve only a few interested individuals. The support for this approach will have to grow and involve more of the health system's most powerful decision-makers before reciprocal communications and participatory relationships become a common practice.

The present organization of many of this country's health facilities is designed for efficiency and cost-effectiveness. As a result, any activities which lengthen the time of a health care visit will be suspect until benefits can be documented. In addition, new financial incentives are needed which will reimburse providers for their efforts to keep people well, capable of caring for themselves, and away from health facilities (except for needed visits). Unfortunately, the active-passive model depicted in Table 1 is the most common communication model in use today because of the fee-for-service payment mechanism.

The third barrier to effective professional-consumer participatory communication arises because communication between members of the health care team have often not been free and open. In fact, for the mutual participation model to work, the style of communication between the members of the health care team will, in many instances, have to change. No amount of encouragement from providers will convince parents and children that they should communicate freely and become involved in their own care if the professionals working within the facility do not seem to have this same privilege.

Education to Overcome Communication Barriers

Having identified certain barriers to two-way communication, the Colorado faculty has redesigned its communication course for school nurses so that these issues are studied in some depth. For example, nurses learn to evaluate the content of their communications with parents and children to see how much of what they say is idle "chit chat" as opposed to meaningful interactions which encourage consumer involvement and learning. While it is true that mutual participation interactions take more time than the active/passive model, it is possible to reduce the time involved by weeding out nonessential conversation.

There are a number of teaching techniques which we have found beneficial in training nurses for reciprocal communication patterns with parents and children. Throughout this paper, I have purposefully referred to the parent and child as health consumers rather than as patients. It is my belief and the belief of our faculty that if nurses are to implement the philosophy that a visit for health care is a joint problem-solving venture, then they must believe that it is appropriate for parents and children to be on more equal footing with professionals. Likening health care visits to other kinds of consumer activities (which involve the selection and purchase of services as well as products) has been an effective way to get this point across. Specifically, our faculty introduces student nurses to the four consumer rights endorsed by Congress in 1964: the right to be heard, the right to be informed, the right to choose, and the right to safety. As these rights are discussed and their implications explored, the rationale for establishing a mutual participation relationship with families and their children becomes abundantly clear.

Perhaps one of the most effective classroom exercises employed to train the nurses to move to a mutual participation model involves having the nurses complete a questionnaire. The Assertive Health Consumer Questionnaire increases their awareness of their own behaviors when they must seek health care for themselves and their families. Below are a few of the items from the questionnaire:

1. When I go to a health care provider, I want him/her to tell me

what to do and how to do it.
2. When I disagree with a health care provider or want another opinion, I always tell him/her directly.
3. It's a mess when I want another medical opinion. I never know how to handle the situation with my own health care provider.
4. I have questions when I see the health care provider, but frequently they don't get asked so they go unanswered.

Once the questionnaires are completed (on a scale of "Most like me" to "Most unlike me"), the discussion begins in earnest. Faculty members help the students move beyond wanting to share every nightmarish experience they, their friends, and family have ever encountered in a health facility. During this process, the nurses usually automatically incriminate physicians as the individuals most responsible for keeping health consumers dependent. At this point, faculty members use examples of nurses' controlling behavior, and help the students focus on their own difficulties in accepting the consumer as a partner in health care. The next phase in this exercise involves identifying the barriers to participatory relationships. Time, lack of administrative support, and personal biases about consumer and provider roles are the barriers most frequently mentioned. The final phase of this classroom activity involves the search for solutions which will eliminate the barriers. One solution which has been very well received is to provide the nurses with specific time management techniques.

As the nurses go through the exercise just described, inevitably another issue that comes up is that of consumer support for reciprocal communications. Most people are more used to active/passive or guidance/cooperation relationships in dealings with health professionals than they are with the mutual participation model. Because of this, the consumer — as well as the nurse — must learn new behaviors.

Consequently, the nurses learn a set of behaviors to teach to consumers (adults and children alike) which will increase consumer participation during visits for health care. These five behaviors are contained in a program called Project Health P.A.C.T. (for Participatory and Assertive Consumer Training).

1. **Tell** about yourself;
2. **Learn-Listen** to new ways to take care of yourself;
3. **Ask** questions;
4. **Decide** what to do jointly; and
5. **Do** follow-up on your own health.

The evaluation of the effectiveness of this nursing training approach is currently underway. Preliminary reports from nurses and parents indicate that the nurses are actually transferring what they have learned in the classroom to clinical settings, and that more reciprocal relationships are emerging. It may well be that this training program — which focuses on health consumerism, what it is like to be a health consumer, and specific ways to enhance communication during visits for health care (rather than focusing on the theoretical aspects of the communication process) — has merit.

I'd like to make two final points regarding this training program for nurses. First, Colorado faculty members feel strongly that the scope of communication training should be multidisciplinary, and that professionals and consumers should be trained together. Second, given the stereotypes that people develop as they age, this kind of training belongs in nursing, medical, and dental schools so that students are able to use mutual participation communication models with health consumers and other professionals from the beginning of their training.

Finally, because childhood is the most teachable moment, nurses must be educated to teach self-responsibility and an active health consumer role to children.

DISCUSSION

Lee Schorr: I want to ask a question although I do not know whether Joy feels she can speak for Judy Igoe. I understand from Judy's paper that the active participation of the consumer is a goal that should be striven for in every relationship. Does everybody agree on that, or are there people for whom the mutual participation model is inappropriate?

Joy Penticuff: I think that your intrepretation of Judy's work is correct. In my own view, there are incompetent people for whom mutual participation as a goal may not be realistic. This may sound quite prejudiced, but I think it is a reality of life.

Mary Ann Lewis: I agree. I think there are people for whom such a model is inappropriate, and I think there are many people who do not want to participate. They want us to tell them what to do and, if we accept the burden, then it becomes our problem.

Bob Chamberlin: I think there is a cultural value involved with the mutual participation model. Most cross-cultural psychiatric studies that I know of have reached the conclusion that as long as a patient and the therapist share the same belief system, you get about the same results no matter what interaction model you use. And I would suspect that this finding would apply to the mutual participation model as well.

Andy Selig: What I tried to say in my presentation, and what I think most of us have said in many different ways, is we agree that professionals have to try to interact with patients, but that for some people the mutual interaction model would not be appropriate.

Lee Schorr: But Judy's paper goes a little further than that. She seems to be saying that it is up to the professional to decide where patients should be going, and that is to the mutual participation model. I guess I may be uncomfortable because it may not be appropriate for the professional to make the judgment that the patient's goal is the wrong goal.

Earl Schaefer: But if we want the patient to be interested in his or her own health care outside of the health care setting, doesn't that patient have to have initiative, decisiveness, and intrinsic motivation? How do you develop those traits unless it is in a mutual participatory monologue, talking with the patient about the self-learning, listening, asking questions, deciding, and following through? It seems to me it is almost essential that we try to develop the mutual participation model, even though we will not succeed with all people.

Joy Penticuff: I agree with you, but I guess I am thinking about our earlier discussion about the people in our society who really are not capable of independent functioning. Although I see them as a very small minority, I think that in nursing we have a tendency to have some extremely fine ideas and to overgeneralize. I think that you have to look at each case individually.

Chuck Lewis: We should all keep in mind that we as health professionals and involved parents frequently overestimate the importance of health to the majority of individuals. I have seen data which suggest that health really is not that big a deal to many. Bleeding is a big deal. Being sick is a big deal. But with children, particularly, health is an abstraction that you are trying to sell. I think when someone becomes ill, they probably become motivated about health, and you then may have a teachable moment in which you can move them toward the mutual participation model.

Gus Swanson: The President's Commission on Medicine and Biomedical Research is releasing its report on informed consent, and they are placing great emphasis on the need for shared decision-making by the patient and the professional. They have emphasized this to the point where I think they have lost sight of the fact that a lot of people would rather have decisions made for them. I think you cannot generalize. You cannot say that *all* patients should be forced to share in a decision about whether to have a radical mastectomy or whether to have other treatments. It is a very complex business. I guess I would say that professionals have to assist in every way those patients who wish to share in decision-making.

Joy Penticuff: I think one of the things that Judy's paper brings out is that her program has taught professionals and children specific skills through a very behavioral approach, and it has worked, Perhaps people who are now incapable of active participation will very gladly step into a participation model when there are appropriate techniques, like these, for teaching them.

Chuck Lewis: I will look forward to Judy's study of the long-term effectiveness of P.A.C.T. because of our own experiences. We have been disillusioned by having shown rather immediate gains in children's behavior, but having that followed by nonreinforcement in family situations. It really does not make a lot of sense to teach children decision-making skills that they are unable to use in their environments. All it does is frustrate them, and it also makes the parents angry, leaving them wondering what in the world the schools are doing to their children.

GOALS, ROLES, AND CONTENT OF PARENT-PROFESSIONAL INTERACTION: PARENT EDUCATION AND PARENT SUPPORT

Earl S. Schaefer, Ph.D.

The health, development, and well-being of children are increased through improvements in parental and professional care, and these improvements are influenced by the quantity, quality, and content of parent-professional interactions. This assertion might be disputed by those who would reduce the role of professionals in the lives of families, and by professionals whose goal is to provide care to children without parental involvement. Yet the major role that parents play in child care, and the need to increase the effectiveness of parenting to enhance child development would support my opening statement. I believe that child health will neither be improved by a return to the Age of the Family, in which families had almost sole responsibility for children, nor by unlimited extension of the Age of Professions and Institutions. Instead, we must work toward an Age of Ecology, in which communication, cooperation, and collaboration between parents and professionals will improve the care of children.

Although researchers increasingly recognize the need for effective parent-professional communication, the goals of these interactions are relatively undetermined. Goals to be achieved by communication between parents and professionals include goals for the child, the parents, the family, the professional, the institution, and the program. Goals also vary from the treatment of illness to the promotion of a child's health, development, and well-being. The roles of the professional and of the parent may be partially determined by a number of things, including their expectations, attitudes, values, and skills. Although the issues of goals, roles, and content of parent-child interaction will require detailed analysis, both theory and research may contribute to the search for answers. This search is guided by paradigms that have evolved from past experience. For example, from research on the role of families in child development and from the accumulated experience of child-centered and parent-centered interventions, an ecological perspective on child development has evolved. This perspective emphasizes the child's interaction with the environment, and complements the individualistic perspective that focused upon the isolated child. In the field of health, a biomedical perspective is being supplemented by a biopsychosocial perspective and by increased attention to behavioral and developmental problems. In addition, an emphasis on disease prevention and health promotion is complementing the previous emphasis on treatment of illness. Evidence that an emphasis on development and reinforcement of strengths, skills, and adaptive behavior may be more effective than attempting to screen, diagnose, and treat behavioral problems supports a developmental perspective that complements a pathological perspective in child health.

In short, these emerging perspectives support an ecological paradigm to complement an individualistic paradigm in child health (Table 1). Although the two paradigms must be integrated if we are to have a comprehensive approach to child health, the major focus of this discussion will be on the ecological-developmental paradigm; I will emphasize the promotion of child development by strengthening and supporting family care of the child.

Table 1. Emphasis in Two Perspectives on Child Health That Are Communicated by Health Practice

Questions	Answers	
	The Individualistic, Pathological, Biomedical Perspective	The Socioecological, Developmental, Biopsychosocial Perspective
What are the major child health problems?	Biomedical problems	Behavioral and developmental problems
What is the major goal of health services?	To screen, diagnose, and treat pathology	To foster health and development
Where is child health maintained?	In the health professional's office, clinic, or hospital	In the child's entire life space, particularly in the family
When is child health care provided?	During office, clinic, or hospital visits	During the child's entire life cycle
Who are the health care providers?	Health professionals	Parents and other community members
Who has the most influence upon child health?	Health professionals	Parents
What is the role of the health professional?	To provide direct health care for the child while under the health professional's care	To provide support for the child's care in the family and community

Note—Reprinted from Schaefer, E.S. Professional support for family care of children. In H.M. Wallace, E.M. Gold and A.C. Oglesby (Eds.), *Maternal and child health practices: Problems, resources and methods of delivery* (2nd ed.). New York: John Wiley & Sons, 1982, pp. 433-446.

Goals of Parent-Professional Interaction

Major goals in child health services include the health, development, and well-being of the child. However, a more detailed examination of components of child development might identify more specific goals and objectives. The biomedical focus in child health has emphasized diagnosis and treatment of illness, screening for health problems, and promotion of growth, physical development, and physical health. Increasing concern about behavioral and developmental problems has extended the area of interest to intellectual and social-emotional development.

Health services which are concerned with behavioral and developmental problems must also be concerned with the development of adaptive behavior. Research on teacher ratings of child adaptation has identified three major areas of academic competence and social adjustment: (1) extraversion versus introversion (including sociability and cheerfulness, as opposed to depression and social withdrawal); (2) considerateness versus hostility (with ratings of cooperativeness and obedience, as opposed to conduct problems and resisting control); and (3) academic competence (including verbal intelligence, general intelligence, intrinsic motivation, and curiosity/creativity). A focus on fostering adaptive behavior would complement and partially replace a goal of remediating maladaptive behavior.

With this goal in mind, a major objective of parent-professional interaction might be to support interactions that influence the child's social-emotional and intellectual development. Detailed analyses of parents' interactions with their infants and children have identified patterns of interaction and stimulation, and patterns of educational behaviors by parents which correlate with children's intellectual development. These behaviors include early teaching of academic skills, talking with the child, sharing educational activities, and providing educational experiences and materials in the home and community. My research with Edgerton has also isolated parental child-rearing attitudes, beliefs, and values related to children's academic competence. These findings support an objective of helping parents develop growth-supporting beliefs and values as well as behaviors.

Another area in which research suggests objectives is in patterns of mother-child interaction. Research has shown that interactions of warmth/love/acceptance (as compared with hostility/rejection/neglect) enhance a child's social-emotional adjustment. Dimensions of parental involvement (versus detachment) and lax discipline (versus firm discipline) have also been identified; these vary with the age of the child and have different correlations with child adjustment at different developmental periods. Although further research is needed, early intervention research shows that effective interactions between parents and professionals may contribute to effective interaction patterns between parents and their child.

A number of factors correlate with the intellectual, occupational, and child-rearing competence of parents. These include parental knowledge, skills, and sense of efficacy; perceptions of internal locus of control of his or her life and the life of the child; modern attitudes and beliefs about change and growth; and perceptions and expectations of professions and social institutions. Correlations of parental modernity with child academic competence suggest that professionals who help parents achieve skills and self-direction will also be helping children achieve these goals.

Another area which professionals should consider involves parental relationships. Studies of family relationships and child development find that the quality of mother-father relationships correlates with the social and emotional development of the child. The studies also find that the absence of the father is frequently related to poverty of the mother and child. Therefore, professionals might work to strengthen relationships between a child's mother and father, or relationships with other primary group members (for example, the mother and grandmother).

An ecological perspective suggests that a focus on the isolated child and isolated parent should be complemented by a focus on the family and on the community that provides continuing support. A conceptual analysis of characteristics of family care (Table 2) — as contrasted to professional care — of children identified 10 variables which suggest that the direct influence of professionals on children is less than the influence of the parents. Therefore, I believe that a major goal of the professional should be to strengthen and support family care of the child, and to supplement that care when indicated — but only rarely to supplant family care. Similarly, professionals who wish to assure continuing emotional support for parents might work to strengthen the parents' primary group, rather than to try to supplement or supplant that group.

Professional Roles and Relationships with Parents

An analysis of individuals' relationships with different social groups has identified characteristics of intensity and frequency of interaction, feeling of belonging, physical proximity, and informality of the relationship. Primary group relationships were judged to be high on each of these characteristics, while secondary groups, the modern community, and neighborhood relationships were lower. Relationships between parents and professionals would also be lower than primary group relationships, although this would vary. Achievement of goals in parent-professional interactions would depend upon the expectations and perceptions of roles of both. One role analysis, which attempted to conceptualize possible roles of the professional, is included as Table 3. Dimensions identified were of more equalitarian/reciprocal (versus more hierarchical/nonreciprocal) roles and of close/personal (versus distant/impersonal) roles.

Development of a close, personal relationship would influence the

Table 2. Characteristics of Family Care of the Child

1. **PRIORITY:** Maternal health, nutrition, smoking, and utilization of medical care influence prenatal development. From birth onward, the parents influence the child's nutrition, health care, experiences, and relationships, thus influencing physical health, social and emotional development, and intellectual and academic achievement.

2. **DURATION:** The parents' influence upon the child extends from conception to maturity.

3. **CONTINUITY:** In contrast to the episodic direct care provided by health and education professionals, the parents' care of the child is usually continuous, apart from brief separations.

4. **AMOUNT:** The total amount of health care, both in prevention and treatment, provided by parents is far greater than that provided by health professionals.

5. **SCOPE:** Parents have the opportunity to provide more varied types of care and to share more different experiences and situations with the child than health professionals.

6. **INTENSITY:** The degree of involvement between parent and child, whether that involvement is positive or negative in its effects, is usually greater than the child's involvement with professionals.

7. **PERVASIVENESS:** Parents potentially influence the child's nutrition, home health care, relationships, care from health professions and institutions, and much of the child's total experience that may influence health and development.

8. **CONSISTENCY:** Parents develop consistent patterns of care for the child that have a cumulative effect upon child health and development.

9. **RESPONSIBILITY:** Both the parents and professionals recognize the parents' primary responsibility for the child's health, education, and welfare.

10. **VARIABILITY:** Great variability exists in parental care of children, varying from extremes of parental love and nurturance to extremes of parental neglect and abuse. Great variability exists in parental knowledge, skills, and resources in providing care for the child.

Note—Reprinted from Schaefer, E.S. Professional support for family care of children. In H.M. Wallace, E.M. Gold and A.C. Oglesby (Eds.), *Maternal and child health practices: Problems, resources and methods of delivery* (2nd ed.). New York: John Wiley & Sons, 1982, pp. 433-446.

Table 3. A Matrix of Professional and Parental Roles Generated from Relationship Dimensions

Relationship Dimensions	Close, Personal	Varying	Distant, Impersonal
Democratic/ Equalitarian	Friend/ Friend	Collaborator/ Collaborator	Peer/ Peer
Varying	Intimate/ Intimate	Consultant/ Client	Provider/ Consumer
Authoritarian/ Hierarchical	Parent/ Child	Teacher/ Pupil	Expert/ Layperson

extent to which the professional could provide direct emotional support to the parent and child. Such a relationship might also influence the professional's effectiveness in parent education. This is true although the needs and demands of the parent as well as the role definition and personality of the professional would influence the degree to which warmth and intimacy could be achieved.

The second dimension of democratic/equalitarian (versus authoritarian/hierarchical) roles would also influence the effectiveness of professional support for parents. The expert role of the professional and the layperson role of the parent might contribute to the development of hierarchical, nonreciprocal roles. Yet professional recognition of the importance of parents in the life of the child and of the skills and potentials of parents might contribute to the development of more equalitarian roles. Research on parent-child relationships shows that parents who prefer self-directing values for children, and parents who have progressive, democratic educational and child-rearing attitudes more often rear competent children. Perhaps a goal of parent compliance might change to a goal of promoting parental self-direction in parent-professional relationships. If the parent's initial expectations and needs are for a professional who takes an authoritative role, the professional might encourage the development of a more reciprocal collaborative or peer role. The professional who wishes to increase parental competence might wish to make parents understand the importance of planning and working together to promote child health.

Although I have focused on parent-professional interactions, a similar analysis might identify the role of the professional in parent groups. The professional could be director, leader, lecturer, facilitator, and/or participant in such a group. The rapid growth of such groups — both with and without professional participation — the effectiveness of the groups in providing emotional support and in promoting behavioral change, and the political power of parent groups suggest that professionals should support their development.

The Content of Parent-Professional Interaction

A matrix developed from goals and roles (that is, an analysis of parent-professional interaction), would specify the probable content of communication. If the goal of the health professional who is guided by an individualistic paradigm is to cope with physical illness, and the preferred role is that of a clinician who provides direct care to the child, communication between professional and parent would focus on the child's physical pathology. The focus on physical illness might even exclude attention to behavioral and developmental problems.

In contrast, if the health professional's goal were developed from an ecological, developmental paradigm, the focus might be upon development of child health through supporting family functioning. The content of the interview (Figure 1) might include reinforcing the family's strengths, strengthening primary group relationships, and discussing parental attitudes, values, and behaviors to enhance further growth and development. These steps might increase the parents' sense of efficacy and control, and might also increase their confidence and initiative in primary group relationships. Of course, the responsibility of the health professional for treating and preventing illness as well as for the promotion of health would require an integration of those activities. However, even during care for an illness, the professional with ecological goals would communicate values and behaviors that would contribute to family functioning.

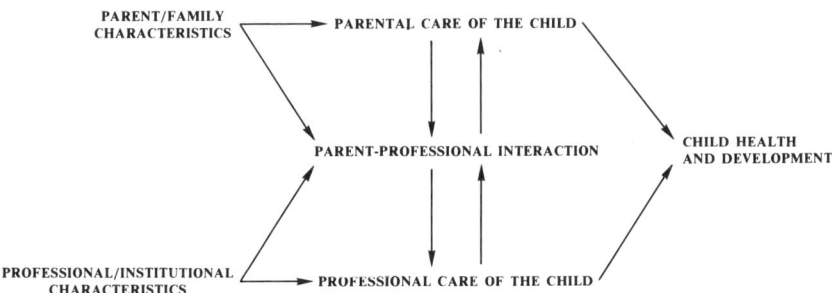

Figure 1. A model for parent and professional care and interaction.

A realistic appraisal of child health services suggests that often health professionals have neither identified developmental goals nor accepted relevant roles in interactions with parents. Few mothers report that they received anticipatory guidance during child health visits in the child's first year of life. In fact, as long ago as 1962, Stine observed little discussion of child behavior or development during pediatric visits. In 1969, Starfield and Barkowf reported that parents' questions were often unacknowledged and unanswered, and in 1974, Chamberlin found that a majority of mothers who felt that their child had behavioral or emotional problems had not talked with a professional about them. Kushner's analysis of the 1981 National Ambulatory Medical Survey suggests that in 80 percent of physician-patient encounters (35 percent self-limited diseases, 35 percent psychosocial problems, and 10 percent preventive services), the clinical model involving diagnosis and treatment is not appropriate. Studies which indicate patient dissatisfaction with medical care and the relatively small need for treatment in office visits have motivated new research investigating the process and content of physician-patient encounters. Patient satisfaction is high when the physician is concerned and willing to listen carefully to the patient's description of symptoms or problems, when the physician gives complete information about their (or their child's) illness and treatment, and when the physician is sensitive to patient and family concerns.

Perhaps current attention to psychosocial factors in child and family health and reports of the positive effects of parent education will encourage interactions between health professionals and parents. A barrier to this may be the reduction of current funding levels for child health programs. Yet researchers, policy makers, and parents have all identified a need for the education of professionals so that the professionals will support family care of children. The need for such education must be addressed if we are to promote the health and well-being of children. The alternative costs — which might include increasing the direct professional care of children or rearing children whose levels of physical health, academic competence, and social adjustment do not allow effective participation in society — are high. The search for fruitful questions, for effective answers, and for funding of parent-professional communication and collaboration must continue.

DISCUSSION

Bob Chamberlin: Earl, our studies did not come up with any clear preference for democratic versus autocratic child rearing. In our study, we followed children from age two into first grade, and using teachers' descriptions, we were unable to distinguish any differences between the children of autocratic and democratic parents. My conclusion was that there are many paths to parenting and there is not any one parenting skill that you can teach that is going to be good for everybody.

Earl Schaefer: I was looking at a low-income sample of families, Bob, while you were essentially looking at middle-class groups. With lower socioeconomic families, we found that self-directing values (which relate to the amount of stimulating interaction the parent gives to the child, whether the parent talks to the child, plays with the child, and praises the child during infancy and the first year of life) do predict the child's competence in kindergarten as described by teachers five years later.

Chuck Lewis: Earl, I do not think anybody would disagree with your proposition that professionals ought to get together with parents. Do you have any specific suggestions or strategies for accomplishing that goal? You know that it is notoriously difficult to modify the behaviors of most adults.

Earl Schaefer: I think Eric Schopler, with his TEACCH program for autistic children in North Carolina, has changed paradigms. What he decided was that parents of autistic children were collaborators in the diagnostic and treatment processes for their children. As a result, he has received tremendous parental support and involvement; the parents went to the state legislature and got a million dollars for a program for autistic children. So I think as we change our paradigm, we will get parents' involvement and support. In another setting, a pediatric practice, Caroline Schroeder is providing consultation to parents. She has found on follow-up that directing parents' attention to the child's positive behavior is one of the best mechanisms for a positive model of child development. By teaching parents that a positive model helps a child adjust and cope, she affected a paradigm change from the pathological concept.

Evan Charney: One of the problems that physicians have is that we often move beween all models of patient involvement, sometimes in the course of a single day. The example of asthma is a very good one: when a child presents in an emergency, you do not want mutual participation. You want somebody who can get an intravenous injection in with the correct dosage, and you want someone who moves very, very quickly. Then you want the physician to shift roles so that emphasis is on counseling and answering questions.

Barbara Korsch: I agree with Evan's last comment because I share his view that we as physicians have to communicate differently in different moments. I think that is one of the strengths of the profession, not a problem; I think that one role enhances the other. In regard to another topic, I think you put two sets of outcome variables into your talk, Earl, and I am not sure that either of them has really been clearly established.

Earl Schaefer: I was discussing emotional support and parent education, and it is true that parent education takes a great investment of time. In fact, it may take more time than the physician can give, and perhaps physicians need to use other personnel in parent education efforts, as Bob Chamberlin has suggested. The reason I believe parent education can make a difference is that I had a tutoring program for children from 15 months until three years of age. We had more than 300 visits with children during that 21-month period, and when they reached three years we had a 17 point IQ difference between them and children in a control group. Phyllis Levinstein, who believed that she could work with parents to increase verbal interactions with their children, demonstrated about the same IQ gain after 30 visits over an eight-month period. In fact, her program had more enduring effects on the child's development than my program.

So it seems far more cost-effective to teach parents to provide effective stimulation for the child than to provide a substitute person to do that stimulation. In addition, we are finding that children in developmental day care from birth onward are still not reaching high levels of achievement without parental involvement. So the power of the professional — whether it is the educator or the childcare worker or the physician — definitely appears to be limited. I think that if we do invest in parent education, we will have a payoff.

Lee Schorr: Just a quick comment. I think that most of us are very persuaded by the core of your argument and just wish that you might leave off a few trimmings in order to make the core more clearly apparent. It is the trimmings that raise the question, not the core. The central message you are giving us is that if professionals do not work with children and their parents, then they are going to miss the boat.

STRATEGIES FOR TRAINING PHYSICIANS IN EFFECTIVE INTERPERSONAL COMMUNICATION SKILLS

J. Larry Hornsby, Ed.D.

Medical educators clearly perceive the importance of the physician-patient relationship in the successful management of the patient, and know that this relationship is dependent upon the effective use of interpersonal communication skills. Today's physicians have readily available advanced technology, but there is an increasing recognition of a need in patient care that cannot be bridged by technology: the need to develop and use effective interpersonal communication skills. For some physicians, these skills come naturally; for others they can be gained only through long years of practice. However these skills are learned, they are essential, for in some situations the quality of care may deteriorate if the physician cannot communicate well.

Communication skills are critical in taking patient histories, performing physical examinations, prescribing medication, educating patients, and influencing patient compliance. History-taking is a part of the basic teaching of all medical schools, and many medical educators today realize that merely asking for information does not always ensure that the physician receives the necessary information. Effective history-taking depends upon the interviewer paying close attention to facilitating communication, instead of just collecting data. Most physicians recognize that a patient's nonverbal communication (for example, physical expressions of pain) yields valuable information during physical examinations. What they may not recognize is that physicians also communicate nonverbally through gestures, postures, tone of voice, touch, and facial expressions.

One aspect of health care — writing prescriptions — seems straightforward, but one study, by Mathews, has reported that 27 percent of patients misunderstood their medication instructions. Another 18 percent misunderstood their treatment or diet instructions, and a total of 54 percent of patients either forgot to tell the physician all their medical problems or forgot other instructions relating to their diagnosis and treatment. One or all of these failures may lead to patient noncompliance and may result in treatment failure. (Interestingly, studies have shown that patient noncompliance is usually underestimated by physicians.) One contributing factor to patient compliance or noncompliance is the physician-patient relationship; that is, how the patient perceives the physician's feelings, as positive or negative, impacts compliance, regardless of whether or not that perception is accurate.

It is important that physicians communicate effectively not only with their patients, but with their colleagues and office staff as well. Ineffective communication can lead to increased rates of staff absenteeism, increased office turnover, negative communication in the office, a tense and anxious work atmosphere, interpersonal conflicts, and overall office stress. Ineffective communications can also lead to a decline in the quality of patient care, office productivity, positive communications, and open and spontaneous communications.

Effective interpersonal communication skills can be identified, measured, and successfully taught in a medical setting. However, the question remains as to how physicians can best be *trained* in the effective use of these skills. Therefore, it is the purpose of this paper to present a plan that emphasizes:

1. When physicians should be trained;
2. How physicians should be trained;
3. What content is appropriate for training; and
4. Who should be involved in training physicians.

When to Train Physicians

Obviously, training in interpersonal communication skills should begin long before medical school. Such training should begin in the home environment, when children are taught to relate to family members and peers, and should continue throughout their education. Teachers of children at all age levels should emphasize not only traditional subject matter, but should also stress social relationship skills as well.

Interpersonal communication skills training is required for some disciplines at the college level (for example, teacher education and psychology); however, premedicine majors frequently omit communication training and concentrate instead on courses that will directly prepare them for medical school admission. We in medical education can do very little about the lack of interpersonal communication skills training the applicant receives prior to entrance into medical school; however, we can change entrance requirements to include a college-level communication skills course. This would let both student applicants and medical educators know the importance we place on such training.

The question of when to train physicians in a medical setting is an easy one to answer but a difficult one to implement. A 1979 survey by Kahn, Cohen, and Jason on the teaching of interpersonal skills in American medical schools found that such skills training is an important part of medical school curriculum. However, most programs (61 percent) directed training to first- and second-year students (preclinical), while 26 percent of the programs offered training to third- and fourth-year students (clinical). Moreover, less than 20 percent of the programs which offered training in the preclinical years included any follow-up of that training. This is unfortunate, for without follow-up training and reinforcement, skills are likely to deteriorate.

Medical School Settings

Interpersonal communication skills training must be integrated at all levels of medical school curricula and across types of training, as follows:

1. Training should begin just prior to the students' first clinical experience. At this point, students are quite receptive to patient care material.
2. Training should be part of every course where students have patient interactions. Technical skills and procedures are reinforced constantly across specialty rotations (for example, history-taking, and diagnostic and management skills); however, communication training is usually a one-shot approach, and is often ignored unless the student is flagrantly deficient in relating to patients. All interaction experiences with patients should provide instructional feedback on the physician-patient process, including its effects on the patient as well as on the student. This continuity of instruction and feedback must be included across clinical specialties, especially during the intensive clinical years.
3. Training should not ignore preceptorships. Not only can the preceptor serve as an excellent role model communicator, but the private practice setting is a good arena for demonstrating the cause and effect of effective physician-patient interactions. In addition, because preceptors usually deal with only one student at a time, they are able to provide one-to-one instructional feedback and reinforcement of communication skills which have

been learned previously.
4. Electives in interpersonal communication skills training may be offered just prior to ward rotations. Such electives should be restricted to a small number of students (ideally six to 12), and are best taught in an outpatient setting. Students, who are eager for patient contact, are also eager to learn practical skills in relating to patients. In addition, learning how to relate well to patients may help prepare students to manage "ward rotation anxiety."

Residency Training Settings

Instructional continuity must be stressed during residency training as well as during medical school education. Even though residents may not have had adequate interpersonal communication skills training as undergraduates their interpersonal skills can be improved in residency programs. In fact, residencies can provide a model training environment for communication training for several reasons. Residencies often have a more desirable faculty-resident ratio, offer faculty members constant exposure to the students for three or more years, have a variety of faculty members, and can set aside time for interpersonal communication skills training. Additionally, many primary care residencies (such as those in family practice and pediatrics) have behavioral science faculty available for communication skills training. However, interpersonal communication skills training should occur in all specialties, not just in primary care specialties.

Although residents are (unfortunately) frequently stressed to learn required curriculum, manage difficult patients, and prepare for board certification, most are open to improving or learning relationship skills that will facilitate effective physician-patient interactions. Of course, faculty of the resident's specialty should assume primary responsibility for shaping the resident's interpersonal communication skills; emphasis must be placed on all resident-patient/family interactions, as well as on resident-staff interactions.

Private Practice Settings

Physicians in private practice are besieged with difficult and complex patient (individual and family) management problems, as well as interpersonal and organizational office conflicts. Despite these many pressures, continuing medical education courses in interpersonal communication skills are generally well received. This is true because many private practitioners see the need and practical uses for interpersonal communication skills. In fact, physicians seem to take such courses depending on the need they perceive for it, regardless of their years in practice. During the last nine years, I have conducted many such courses, and frequently have been asked, "Why didn't they teach me this in medical school and residency training?" In all probability, interpersonal communication skills training may have been offered; but the physician may not have been receptive at that time, may not have received instructional continuity, or may have had ineffective role models. Thus, continuing medical education courses may be the last chance for many physicians to learn interpersonal communication skills.

How to Train Physicians

A number of surveys illustrate the wide variety of methods used to teach interpersonal communication skills in medical settings, but research studies show that one method is only marginally more effective than another. Unfortunately, most studies have focused on interviewing skills, and not primarily on interpersonal communication skills; nevertheless, the question of how to teach physicians must be addressed.

Medical Students

The following questions must be answered by those selecting teaching methodologies for medical students:

1. How can the students best acquire cognitive knowledge?
2. How can cognitive attitudes best be altered?
3. How can skills implementation and practice best be designed?
4. How can instructional feedback best be provided?
5. How can evaluation (by faculty and self) best be provided?
6. How can instructional continuity and follow-up training and reinforcement best be ensured?

In answering these questions, medical educators must also consider such traditional issues as identifying subject content and teaching faculty, securing curriculum time, determining class or course size, and selecting physical facilities for a course. Naturally, answers to the six questions will vary widely, and an interpersonal communication skills training program that is successful at one school may fail at another. Nevertheless, the following four approaches represent the most widely used instructional methods in teaching interpersonal communication skills.

1. One method involves the use of self-instructional or programmed manuals. This step-by-step method is most successful for use outside the classroom, and supplements other teaching methods. Outside preparation saves in-class time, allows students to work at their own pace, and helps prepare students to make best use of class time. When this method is selected, it is important that a feedback component be included to evaluate each student's progress. Examples of such a feedback component include self-instructional manuals, programmed videotapes and slide-tapes, and interactive films.
2. Another instructional method involves small group seminars. Such seminars allow greater teaching flexibility due to fewer numbers of students. They generally involve a combination of mini-lectures with skills development and practice. Practice sessions may include video "trigger" tapes, role-play situations, live demonstrations, simulated patient interactions, and real patient encounters. Small group seminars may be used as a subcomponent of large lecture classes.
3. A third instructional method involves lectures. Whether in large or small group settings, lectures are simply inadequate unless they are supplemented by other methods. When teaching interpersonal communication skills, it is critical that a skills development and practice component be included; otherwise the communication training lectures become "just another course," to be forgotten along with the other nonessential courses.
4. A fourth instructional approach is modeling. Students can learn effective interpersonal communication skills by observing the actions of faculty role models. Naturally, all faculty should serve as good role model communicators when interacting with patients, students, or other colleagues. Unfortunately, this is frequently the exception rather than the rule, for faculty often become preoccupied with demonstrating technical skills and procedures and may ignore the communication process. Since modeling effects will occur whenever faculty members are working with a patient in front of students, it is critical that the faculty be very selective about their behavior.

A creative faculty member should be able to use any combination of instructional methods when focusing on interpersonal communication skills training. The critical aspects of teaching communication skills includes making sure that students acquire basic communication concepts, that they are allowed to practice communication skills while receiving helpful feedback, and that faculty members — regardless of their clinical specialty — reinforce the physician-patient communication process continually throughout all clinical rotations.

Residents

Residency training programs are an excellent arena for systematically teaching interpersonal communication skills, for faculty members have the opportunity to closely observe and shape the resident's behavior over a period of three to four years.

In residency programs, communication skills training should emphasize practical applications in both inpatient and outpatient clinics. Videotaped feedback of residents working with their own patients is the method of choice, although other methods may be used as needed. The use of videotapes allows residents to develop and/or improve their interpersonal communication skills by: (1) sharpening their ability to understand what patients are saying both verbally and nonverbally; and (2) changing their own verbal and nonverbal behavior to create more effective communication with patients.

A systematic approach to training, continuous constructive feedback by faculty members, and self-evaluation should be undertaken throughout the resident's training, especially during their chosen specialty rotations. Role modeling and continuous reinforcement — regardless of the type of patients or clinical procedures — are essential to produce effective physician communication.

Private Practitioners

Continuing medical education courses are the major means of developing and reinforcing private practitioners' interpersonal communication skills. The workshop approach (which permits concentrated time for skills acquisition and practice, evaluation, and implementation in private practice) appears to be the most successful method. Physicians who attend such workshops are eager to learn different ways of communicating with their patients and staff. Self-instructional programs, usually via correspondence courses, are sometimes used, but these are generally less than effective because they do not permit practice under expert supervision.

Home-site implementation should include ways that the physician can receive regular feedback regarding their interpersonal communication skills from patients and their office staff.

Appropriate Content for Training

In order for physicians to be effective communicators, they must possess basic interpersonal communication skills concepts, a way to communicate these concepts, and an understanding of patients' age-related behavior.

Basic Interpersonal Communication Skills Concepts

Empathy, respect, warmth, concreteness, genuineness, and self-disclosure are the interpersonal skills needed to develop positive relationships, establish physician-patient rapport, and establish an atmosphere of trust, cooperation, and mutual respect in the medical setting. Research has indicated that training in these specific areas has been used successfully to improve interpersonal communication skills in settings such as medicine, allied health, dentistry, industry, teacher education, penal institutions, and city and state governments.

Vehicle for Communicating Interpersonal Communication Skills

The medical interview is where interpersonal communication skills and medical training merge. Gathering information, evaluating it, discussing the findings with patients, and planning and monitoring treatment all depend on the interview. Interpersonal communication skills and medical interviewing are not synonomous, and it should not be assumed that all physicians receive training in interviewing techniques, although they all do receive training in history-taking. Therefore, physicians need to learn specific interviewing techniques; these include how to open and close an interview, how to ask questions to elicit and restrict information, and how to ask questions in such a way that the physicians can use their clinical acumen. At the same time, physicians should demonstrate effective interpersonal communication skills while conducting the medical interview. Both interpersonal communication skills and interviewing skills are learned behaviors that should be systematically emphasized throughout medical training.

Age-Related Patient Behavior

Since children are the focus of this Round Table, I would like to mention pediatric age-related behavior at this point. When communicating with children, the physician must demonstrate the following understanding and abilities.

1. A working knowledge of child growth and development concepts that include physical, cognitive, sexual, and psychosocial aspects is essential. Developmental and behavioral tasks for

each stage of development should be emphasized.
2. An understanding of the common behavioral problems of childhood and their effects on the child and family is essential.
3. An attitude of patience, tolerance, acceptance, and encouragement for both the child and family should be communicated.
4. The physician must have the ability to provide an open and nonthreatening atmosphere.
5. The child must be accepted as an active participant in the physician-child/family interaction. Of course, such participation depends on the child's cognitive level and ability to understand and communicate effectively.
6. The physician must demonstrate the ability to facilitate communications with the child through interpersonal communication skills, drawings, touch, toys, anatomy models, and so forth.
7. Skills in balancing communication with the child and the parents, without ignoring either, are essential.

Addressing the Question of Who Should Train Physicians

What type of faculty is most frequently used to provide interpersonal communication skills training? A 1979 study by Kahn et al. reported that physicians, psychiatrists, internists, family physicians, and pediatricians are (respectively) the most frequently used teachers for communication skills training. Psychologists, social workers, and medical sociologists are used most frequently as trainers among nonphysicians, while psychiatrists and psychologists are used most frequently among both groups. I am not aware of any research that demonstrates superiority among disciplines or specialties in teaching interpersonal communication skills.

Since physicians have the primary responsibility for educating other physicians, it is natural (and indeed recommended) that they assume the greater role in providing interpersonal communication skills training in the medical setting. That physicians have a clear advantage over nonphysicians in fully integrating interpersonal communication skills training with technical skills and procedure is axiomatic. Physicians also have more exposure to students and residents, which provides a greater opportunity for continuity of instruction and continuous reinforcement throughout medical training.

Should nonphysicians play an important role in interpersonal communication skills training for physicians? The answer, although it is probably biased, is yes. As a rule, nonphysicians have had more extensive interpersonal communication skills training and have obtained more experience in teaching interpersonal communication skills to many different medical specialties and disciplines. Many physicians have had little or no direct interpersonal communication skills training in their medical education, so physician faculty members may not be prepared to systematically provide communication skills training. Therefore, nonphysicians may provide development courses in interpersonal communication skills to physician faculty members who may later provide interpersonal communication skills training to students and residents.

Physicians and nonphysicians should work together to plan, develop, implement, and evaluate interpersonal communication skills training. Initially, intensive training should be co-taught by physicians and nonphysicians. Later, it is probably best for the nonphysician to function in a consultant role as needed.

DISCUSSION

Gus Swanson: Larry, you commented that medical schools should consider requiring courses in interpersonal communication skills. I would argue against adding any more course requirements, partly because medical schools are the only schools educating professionals that so strongly steer the curriculum of students. In fact, right now I am arguing that we should give up fixed course requirements in physics, chemistry, and biology. My basic philosophic reason for doing this is that I do not think we should arrogantly dictate what students who are responding to medicine can study.

Larry Hornsby: Some people would add to your argument by asking if all medical students and residents really need communication skills training. In fact, many medical students do not need such training. Some of them walk in with great skills. Yet it seems that those who need such training too often do not get it. I guess the point I am trying to make is that if medical schools require a certain level of communication skills for entrance, then communication skills courses will be seen as extremely important and not just another course.

Mary Ann Lewis: But, Larry, while it is true that those who come with good skills may not need communication training, my experience is that they really do not know *why* they are good communicators. So I would argue that even students who communicate well need training. Having said that, I would like to ask what you see as the barriers to teaching communication skills to medical students.

Larry Hornsby: From looking at a number of different medical schools, I have come to believe that they choose the wrong faculty members to teach communication skills courses. In addition, the courses are not allowed enough time. The courses are taught in the first quarter, and often there is no patient care experience until the second year; in that period, communication has become a forgotten skill. Also, there is really no reinforcement of good communication throughout the four years. Most medical schools at least attend to some aspect of communication skills training in the first or second year, but by the third and fourth years when students are really seeing patients on the wards, it is a forgotten field.

Jim Strain: I think Larry's point about role modeling is excellent, and I want to reemphasize it. I see faculty members communicating well with the chief resident and secondary resident but not relating to the patients very well. They tell the first year resident, for example, to go talk to the family about a problem and then report back. I think we need to emphasize to all faculty members that they really have a great deal to offer by talking directly with the patients while the residents are present and observing.

Chuck Lewis: Getting back to what we all seem to agree is one of the major issues, we have no good instruments for either selecting applicants for medical school or for determining students' progress. I am currently working with a test committee which is looking at the National Boards, and all I can tell you is it has been a very frustrating experience. When a question tries to capture something other than sociological knowledge, it is thrown out as being too general, or lacking in validity, and so on.

CHILD HEALTH CARE COMMUNICATIONS: PREPARING PHYSICIANS IN TRAINING

Evan Charney, M.D.

Much has been written about communication barriers between

patients and physicians. There are well-documented gaps in the process and abundant public testimonial to the fact that physicians are often not as sensitive to or skilled at communication as they might be. How can we as professionals address the problem?

A variety of strategies need to be considered, a number of which are being discussed at this conference. They include the following:

1. **Select medical students who give promise that they will be skilled in communication.** I believe that this is the single most important strategy for improving physician communications, since personality and character traits are so well established by the time students enter medical school that subsequent education can only realistically be expected to enhance or diminish them. I realize that making such selections will not be easy. Although it is easier to assess such areas as biochemical competence than to measure empathetic competence, we need to continue to work at the task.

2. **Provide better communication skills training in medical schools.** We in medical education probably expend more of our energies on this strategy than on any of the others I will list. Yet we tend to identify "communication skills" (as well as biochemistry, physiology, and other "basic sciences") as somehow separate from the fabric of clinical practice. Then we are disappointed when our students are unable to integrate this knowledge when they approach a patient's problem.

3. **Provide better training about communication skills in the residency years.** This will be the subject of my talk, and I'll return to it later.

4. **Provide better continuing education for practicing physicians.** We probably do this least well, somehow assuming that communication skills are immutable by the time a physician is in practice, and that adequate skills will not diminish over time. Neither assumption may be correct, of course. Our traditional continuing education models — written materials, audio digest tapes, or the several day "update conference" — are likely to be the least effective educational strategies. The ongoing Balint workshop model for practitioners makes the most sense and has been well described, although it has not been widely utilized. I will consider the place for such a workshop later in this discussion.

The Importance of Teaching Communication Skills During Residency

For the purposes of this conference I will focus on the residency period as a particularly crucial time to learn communication skills for two main reasons. First, residency is a time of great stress, during which there is an enormous acquisition of new skills. Second, there is reason to believe that we are not as successful at teaching interpersonal communication skills as we might be. Mumford refers to the internship as a particularly important "imprinting" period, and the entire residency certainly contains all the ingredients necessary for forging a new professional identity. The subjects are separated from their usual sources of support; are placed in a confined space for long hours (the hospital); are deprived of sleep; are given a considerable number of new responsibilities and skills to learn, often without adequate emotional support; and are expected to display the stoicism and single-minded devotion to patient care characteristic of Rex Morgan, M.D. Little wonder that Valko and Clayton have found that 30 percent of first-year residents suffered from clinical depression, or that the American Medical Association's Department of Mental Health has designated houseofficers as a group at special risk of mental illness. To quote Siegel and Donnelly, who described a support group for pediatric interns at Boston City Hospital:

> Internship may be critical not only because of the impact of the year itself but also for the implicit expectation that this is the way medicine works and that this is how the life of a physician must be. The frequently reported treadmill existence of physicians . . . may in part be a by-product of imposing on oneself the same time demands that were required during residency training.

In the hectic climate of residency, learning effective communication skills is the kind of subject matter likely to be most readily sacrificed. Although psychosocial factors of patient care are no less important than acute care management issues, they *appear* to be less imperative, and can be more easily avoided in the course of a day's work. Werner, Adler, Robinson, and Korsch, in an excellent study of attitudes during pediatric residency, found that residents considered psychosocial factors and physician-patient relationships less important as a determinant of illness and effective patient care following their internships than at the beginning of the year. I believe that observation to be both important and valid, and also of great concern, for residents' performance and attitudes at the completion of residency are very predictive of how they will behave during at least the first years of their practice life.

If we grant that the residency years are precious ones for developing attitudes and skills in communication, and that these skills are not always learned as well as they could be, how can we address the issue?

Developmental Stages of Residency

Brent has written a perceptive article in which he suggests that we consider the residency as a developmental process. Drawing on the work of Levinson and colleagues on adult developmental stages and Zaborenko and Zaborenko on medical students, Brent proposes that medical residents need to negotiate a number of conflicts. These are as follows.

1. **Vulnerability-Invulnerability.** Young physicians struggle with their own feelings of inadequacy and their patients' expectations of an omnipotent, invulnerable healer. Residents vacillate between these feelings, sometimes in the course of a single day. As they develop a core of competence, the residents are better able to tolerate vulnerability in themselves, their colleagues, and their patients.
2. **Active-Passive.** The physician's need to be active and in control conflicts with the realities of chronic disease and complex psychosocial factors. Residents are led to believe that, with enough knowledge and skill, disease can be controlled, and senior residents and faculty members often behave as if that is the case. Unfortunately, the reality is that many patients cannot be cured — they can only be comforted and supported.
3. **Helplessness-Problem Solving.** Placed in a situation where the complexities of illness, poverty, and the social organization of the hospital are seen as unfair barriers to the ability to "cure," residents may withdraw and complain. Until the residents grasp that they are part of the system and learn how to negotiate in the hospital environment, they may not be able to successfully address this conflict. It is evident that many physicians do not ever resolve the conflict either. These physicians have concluded that problems of patient compliance and the psychological and social factors of illness are outside their own professional role. As physicians, we become skilled at avoiding situations we're unlikely to do well in, but the residents have no such option.
4. **Boundary Maintenance.** Zaborenko refers to the dichotomy of "objectivity and empathy," where the resident's task is to determine how close he or she can get to other staff members and patients without abandoning the professional role. At another level, this "boundary" refers to the line between personal life and work. Physicians in training need to locate themselves somewhere between the uncommitted, self-indulgent physician and

the "workaholic" researcher or clinician who never leaves the laboratory or the hospital.
5. **Professional Identity.** The developmental tasks listed above are perhaps summed up by this one, which is the consolidation of the resident's professional identity. Residency is a time to fashion an identity based on observations of various mentors and role models and on receiving adequate and timely feedback.

I have presented this developmental format because the strategies for teaching communication skills are very much influenced by an understanding of the conflicts the resident faces. Residents cannot attend to the affective and attitudinal parts of their development without considerable support and modeling from their teachers. I'll outline two main strategies and briefly consider each: support programs for pediatric residents and teaching communication skills by faculty role models.

Strategies for Residency Training Programs

A variety of support efforts have been employed in residency programs. Berg and Garrard found this when they surveyed 481 residency program directors in six medical specialties, and reported on the frequency and types of support offered to residents. Table 1 lists their findings for all the specialty groups combined and separately for pediatrics and family practice. In general, family practice and psychiatry programs were found to more often provide psychosocial support services. The study does not consider whether the residents in the program thought that these services were helpful, of course, but it does indicate the spectrum of support services available. The point here is that faculty members ought to carefully consider such programs. Providing residents with psychosocial support — faculty-resident communication — is tangible evidence that we treat residents as whole persons, just as we advise them to do with their own patients.

Support group efforts in pediatrics have included retreats of one or more days in which the subject of patient-doctor communication is discussed, and ongoing resident discussion groups led by department pediatric faculty and/or mental health counselors. Both Siegel and Strahilevitz make the useful observation that such group sessions first need to let residents list their complaints about the stress and fatigue of the program before they proceed to a discussion of coping mechanisms.

I would add that a residency program should have an identified faculty advisor for each resident. This faculty person should serve a

Table 1. Psychosocial Support Programs for Residents*

	All Programs (n–481)	Family Practice (n=88)	Pediatrics (n=81)
Support Groups	40	59	37
Part-Time Residency	24	13	25
Professional Counselors	66	83	65
Child Care Services	9	7	6
Formal "Gripe" Sessions	80	90	77
Seminars:			
Medical Issues	78	93	84
Personal/Professional Issues	36	72	19
Paid Sick Leave	94	93	93
Social Activities	88	91	94
Financial Advisor	25	57	20

*Berg and Garrard, 1980

role separate from that of the chief resident (the foreman) or the chairman or residency program director (the boss). The advisor should obtain feedback about the resident's performance on each rotation (including observations by nursing and support staff) and should regularly discuss that information with the resident. This faculty advisor should not be a psychotherapist (if clear counseling needs are identified, special help must be sought); in effect, the advisor plays the role of the generalist physician to the resident, and serves as his or her advocate in the program. It may be useful for those selected for the advisory role (and not every faculty member will be appropriate) to meet as a group to define their goals and methods and to consider pertinent issues. Although providing organized feedback to residents (via faculty advisors and other methods) is now clearly mandated as a requirement by the Accreditation Council for Graduate Medical Education of the American Medical Association, many faculty advisor programs are not as thoroughly developed as they might be.

Finally, I should like to stress the importance of patient-doctor communication skills being modeled throughout the residency by faculty members. In particular, such modeling should be done by those responsible for teaching primary care pediatrics. A psychiatric liaison service is certainly helpful, as are designated behavioral rounds, lectures, or seminar series on communication topics. However, if residents learn that communication skills are a *special* topic taught by *special* staff at a *special* time, they may well conclude that it is permissible not to consider the subject at other times. Communication skills are better demonstrated than discussed, and must be part of the warp and woof of daily clinical rounds.

An example of the importance of such modeling involved the case of a first-year pediatric resident. The resident was faced with counseling the family of a one-year-old child who had suffered irreversible brain damage in an accident and was being considered for withdrawal from ventilator support. The family had no primary physician, and had developed close ties with the resident during the time the child was hospitalized. The faculty advisor sat with the resident and the family as the child's condition was reviewed, and added his own comments to the discussion; the day following the child's death, the resident and faculty advisor together made a visit to the family's home. The automobile ride out to the home provided an important time for the resident to confide her own feelings of depression and helplessness about the case. In fact, discussing this issue outside of the hospital seemed valuable in itself. At first the resident was apprehensive about the home visit, saying that she feared being placed in a situation in which the family rather than the physician would be "in control." From this experience, the resident learned that the physician's presence itself at such times is the really important factor. A supportive and experienced role model was extremely valuable, for it helped the resident through a developmental crisis and allowed the resident to address the professional issues involved in this experience.

As this vignette suggests, it is valuable for the resident to directly observe faculty members interact with families in many ways, including during interviews. Residency programs should find it as important to videotape faculty interviews as resident interviews. In our program, a behavioral workshop for senior residents is conducted twice monthly by a practitioner from the community and a full-time primary care faculty member. These professionals review cases (including their own) to demonstrate to residents that psychosocial management can be an important and satisfying part of clinical practice. I do not mean to demean the role of the subspecialist in teaching communication skills. Indeed, subspecialists often provide residents with the best examples of the "compleat physician" who can attend both to the physiology and psychology of patient care. However, the immediacy and fascination with the biomedical process being considered often occupies the discussion largely or exclusively, relegating communication issues to the afterthought category reserved for the "art of medicine" part of rounds.

It is necessary for faculty who teach communication skills to practice them, of course. That would seem a truism, except that ambulatory faculty often spend so much time with administrative duties that they practice very little or not at all. As with all clinical skills, sensitivity in patient communication does atrophy with disuse. That is why we have found it valuable (and satisfying) in our programs to encourage an ongoing workshop on patient management problems in the behavioral area for faculty members and several practitioners. The sharing of problems during the workshops may include direct interviewing of a family or the review of audio- or videotapes, and can be extremely helpful. The workshop group is composed of 10 members who meet twice monthly for a two-hour evening session built around a case presentation. All participants are pediatricians; five are full-time faculty members, and five are in pediatric practice and have significant involvement in resident education. Four of the group members also have had fellowship training in behavioral and developmental pediatrics.

At a recent meeting a pediatric practitioner sought the group's advice for the following case: Both parents of a five-year-old child under the physician's care had been killed in a double homicide four weeks earlier. The father had stabbed the mother to death, and had in turn been shot by the mother's sister. The five-year-old girl, who had not witnessed the scene directly and who had not attended the funeral, was currently living with her maternal grandmother and aunt. The grandmother sought help from the pediatrician with a number of specific questions: What should the child be told, beyond the fact that both parents were "in heaven?" How should the grandmother respond to the child's wish to see the parents? What should the school be told? How should the family cope with the child's regressed and demanding behavior? The discussion of this tragic case touched on the five-year-old's concept of death and the role of the pediatrician as counselor and advocate. Of equal importance, the session provided valuable emotional support for the physician, for whom the case raised important issues of helplessness, problem-solving, and boundary maintenance.

At another session, one participant wished to discuss his role as a faculty advisor to an intern who had withdrawn from the program because of psychological decompensation after four months. He wished to ask whether the resident's problems could have been better identified and managed. The group process provoked discussion about the advisory system in the program, and provided important support to the advisor. In other words, this kind of workshop can be considered a working model of continuing education for physicians in practice and in residency teaching programs.

The housestaff is aware of this ongoing workshop, and several have commented that they would like to be involved in such a group themselves when in practice. The clear message intended — and conveyed — by such a workshop is that communication skills are not learned at any one point in medical education, and that they must be continually sharpened throughout a physician's career.

DISCUSSION

Andy Selig: It seems to me you made some very good points about the atmosphere of medical education. But I would like to add a comment. Most physicians' practice in clinical settings is routine care, and anywhere from 30 to 80 percent psychosocially related. Why, then, do training programs for physicians and pediatricians spend such a small proportion of time on psychosocial issues? It seems that the majority of training time is spent on issues that occupy a small proportion of primary care physicians' actual time in practice.

Evan Charney: I think that is a fair comment. In defense of pediatrics, I think there have been changes in the pediatric programs over the past decade, but also I think pediatrics still has a terrific identity crises. Pediatrics still is not sure what it wants to be. Do we want to be hospital-based consultants or do we want to be primary care practitioners? I believe that we struggle with this dichotomy, which is part of the problem. If there is a strong commitment to do both, one thing or another suffers, and I am afraid that the primary care aspects of the curricula are still less well attended to than the consultant aspects.

Jim Strain: I share some of your concern. I really do not think we train residents to practice primary care. What we do is assume that pediatricians are going to deliver primary care, yet we do not always train them that way. The Task Force on Pediatric Education developed an excellent paper about three years ago in which they pointed out that we do not give pediatric residents enough training in the area of ambulatory medicine. Out of that Task Force's report grew some concern among training program directors, and we have seen some shift into providing psychosocial training. However, one of the big problems is that pediatric training programs are often designed to meet service needs in hospitals. The hospital pays for the resident to serve in the newborn nursery, for example. It does not pay for the resident to spend time in a physician's office. I think that many medical training program directors would be very willing to incorporate more ambulatory experiences into the training program if there were some way to fund them. I think that most medical educators would like to provide more experience for residents in the ambulatory care setting in the hospital, and would like to see more continuity clinics.

They would also like to see pediatric residents in pediatricians' offices because I think that is where they learn the communication skills to deal with common practice problems.

Gus Swanson: I think one of our major problems is bringing back emphasis on the development of the basic, fundamental skills that physicians need. Faculty members, who evaluate students as they progress through the four years of medical school and then residency, are putting 95 percent of their emphasis on cognitive evaluation; they are very uncomfortable about evaluating fundamental skills or about taking any action against students who lack those skills. For example, if a fourth-year student who had already masked into the pediatric training program scored 750 on the National Boards in the pediatric section but was judged by faculty to have poor interpersonal skills, would that student be held back? Would some corrective action be taken? I think you would have a hard time convincing the faculty at large that such a step was necessary because the National Board score was high. That is the weight that is placed on the Boards.

Another point I would like to make is about residency training. I have heard residents complaining about the long hours they spend in the hospitals. Those of us who were in residency programs 30 or 40 years ago spent as much time in the hospital as our residents do today. But I have been struck by the fact that the quality of the time spent is quite different. Our residents today are overwhelmed by technological procedures and by making decisions that we did not have to make as residents some years ago. I think that is something we have to take into account as we develop residency programs. We have an environment now which is extremely stressful, and it will not be easy to assist residents simply by providing counseling or group sharing. I think we have to do more than that. We really have to look at the structure of training programs and at the balance between service and the educational progression of residents.

Bob Pantell: Gus has raised some important issues. He has mentioned the emphasis that is placed on the National Boards. I would like to note just how cognitively grounded those Boards are. They pay very little attention to psychosocial skills. The residents know that the Boards they must pass are going to be cognitively grounded, and I think it is easy for them to dismiss a lot of our psychosocial training efforts as a result.

Barbara Korsch: I think this business of evaluation is terribly important. When we started audio- and videotaping residents, what we found sometimes stunned the faculty. We learned that someone could get through our whole system without anyone ever having seen them talk to or examine a patient.

Also, I would like to defend the National Boards for a minute. Developers of the Boards have made an effort through the years to devise an appropriate way of evaluating residents' communication skills. In fact, they once asked us to develop a videotape designed to test sensitivity to interpersonal skills which could be included as part of the examination process. We worked on that tape and we tried to develop some standards, but we never felt comfortable about having it become part of the examination. It is just very difficult to evaluate psychosocial skills.

PART III
TECHNIQUES FOR IMPLEMENTATION: CURRENT POSITION AND FUTURE OPPORTUNITIES

Problems with the ways that physicians and nurses are trained, problems in the way that private pediatrics is practiced, and changes which are needed in health care systems and financing: All these topics were discussed during the third portion of the Round Table.

August Swanson summarizes the status of current medical education programs in the United States, including the numbers and sizes of the programs and how their curricula have evolved. Swanson sees a problem in the "intensive emphasis on detailed memorization of a massive body of facts," stating that this emphasis places great demands on students and detracts from their learning of effective communication skills. He outlines other problems as well, and notes that an advisory panel of the American Association of Medical Colleges believes that many of these problems will not only continue, but will probably become even more pronounced as the technological explosion continues in medicine.

Student nurses, like medical students and residents, are under increasing stress because of the ever-growing volume of information to be learned, according to Joy Hinson Penticuff. Having surveyed American nursing school programs for the Round Table, Penticuff believes that nurses frequently receive more training in psychosocial and communication skills than physicians. However, she says, student nurses are too often being prepared to practice medicine in ways that do not exist in the "real world," a dilemma which leads to disillusionment and professional burnout.

Karen Fond, who discusses the training of nurse practitioners, believes that the nurse practitioner model has "restored nursing's involvement with patients." She describes nurse practitioners' innovative work with children, with mothers, with parent groups, and in teaching and research.

James Strain offers the perspective of a practicing physician in an ambulatory setting. He suggests some ways that practicing pediatricians can communicate effectively with children and families, outlines some strategies for teaching communication skills to physicians, and states his belief that practicing pediatricians can be valuable preceptors for pediatric residents. He notes that pediatrics is a high-volume practice, which adds to the potential for communication problems.

Strain's emphasis on the need to change the financial incentives for practicing physicians was reinforced by Lisbeth Bamberger Schorr, who summarized and put into perspective many recurrent themes of the Round Table. She comments on structural barriers related to public policy which prevent effective communication, and suggests that categorical advocacy groups should join together to broaden their bases of concern. Schorr also urges health professionals to actively be involved in advocating for improved child health.

Susan M. Thornton, M.S.

ACADEMIC TRAINING/ MEDICAL EDUCATION

August G. Swanson, M.D.

Today I'd like to discuss recommendations made by the Association of American Medical Colleges regarding the education of physicians. But first, so that you will understand some of the difficulties we face when we attempt to change that education, I'd like to describe the current medical education system in this country. As of June of 1982, there were 127 medical schools in the United States. They range in class size from more than 300 in Indiana to 50 at the Mayo Clinic School of Medicine. The ages of these institutions vary from the University of Pennsylvania, which was founded in the late 18th century, to Mercer, which was founded in 1982.

There are now 48,000 full-time faculty members in these medical schools, which compares with about 9,000 in 1960. Thirty-six thousand of these faculty members are in clinical departments, while the others are in the basic sciences.

The vast increase in faculty members during the last 15 years has accompanied an expansion in the number of students being admitted to and graduated from medical school. In 1981, we admitted 16,644 students to medical school, which was about one admission per every two applicants. That compares with 1974, 1975, and 1976, when we had 2.8 applicants per position through the United States. One interesting indicator of potential trends is that the Association of American Medical Colleges' Division of Student Services estimates that 16,567 students will be admitted in 1982. That means we will have 77 fewer new entrants to medical school this year than last, which is the first time that there's been a decline in enrollments since the late 1950s. The upward curve may be breaking as far as future expansion in enrollment is concerned.

The medical schools in this country use the resources of 418 major teaching hospitals and an almost uncountable number of ancillary teaching hospitals in one way or the other. Thus you can see that medical education is a large and complex enterprise.

Evolution of Curricula in Medical Schools

During the last decade, there has been relatively little curricular innovation in American medical education. In the 1960s there was a flurry of change and experimentation. In 1961, the first so-called six-year program was developed at Northwestern as a subset program of the medical school. The program called for the selection of very promising students. They were admitted to medical school upon entrance to college, and graduated six years later. This approach spread during the 1960s and early '70s, so that today 12 schools offer a six-year program. The six-year approach and many other curricular changes in the '60s led students to early decision-making regarding the specialty that they would follow, and early tracking of students into their chosen specialties was a feature of many curricular changes.

One major change that occurred during the 1960s was that the senior year in almost all institutions became a totally elective year. Another feature of the 1960's revolution was a reduction in the time students spent in basic science laboratories (physiology, biochemistry, pharmacology, and anatomy), and a vast increase in the number of hours spent listening to lectures.

During the 1970s, the only major curricular innovation was caused by the Congress of the United States. In 1971, Congress passed the Health Professions Educations Act, which offered a bonus to schools that reduced their curriculum to three years. Congress reasoned that this would vastly increase the number of doctors being graduated in the United States. Eighteen schools did attempt to serve the will of the Congress over the period from 1972 through 1978; then they retreated to the more traditional four-year program. Today we have no three-year programs left from that experiment.

Current Medical Education Program

Current programs in American medical schools are characterized by an intense emphasis on the detailed memorization of a massive body of facts. The demands placed on students, particularly during the preclinical years, have grown steadily during the last decade. There has been approximately a one-percent-per-year increase in hours spent in class, so that today, on the average, medical students are spending 30 to 40 hours in class per week. As you know, those 30 to 40 class hours must be balanced by a lot of private study time, which really leaves very little time for thought or for contemplation. The increase in the number of lectures is compounded by the fact that the lectures are given by what students have come to term a "parade of stars." The lectures are being presented by individuals who give only one or two lectures to the class each year, and who take that opportunity to impart their full body of information. The intensity of rather poorly coordinated, in-depth lectures is a cause for complaint by students in most schools.

To further compound the emphasis on detailed memorization of facts, medical school faculties have developed an exceedingly high level of dependence on the National Board of Medical Examiners' three-part, multiple-choice examination system. The first part of the examination covers basic science areas; it consists of 1,000 items and is usually taken by students at the end of their second year. The second part of the examination is about the same length and emphasizes clinical disciplines; it is usually taken just prior to graduation. The third portion, which emphasizes patient management, is taken by most students during their first graduate year. This year, 78 percent of all medical schools in the United States are requiring that their students take the first part of the National Board Examination. In about half of these schools, passing the examination is either required for promotion, or the actual examination scores are used for final course grades. About 72 percent of the schools require students to take the second portion of this examination. I mention the heavy emphasis on this examination because I think it's one of our great problems. While many medical educators talk about trying to produce well-rounded students who have high levels of skill in a whole variety of areas, testing of those skills involves only seeing how much a student can "spill back" on a national multiple-choice examination.

The clinical clerkships are a source of concern to those who would educate physicians to be effective communicators. In almost every medical school, the junior year involves a sequence of required clerkships. On the average, this means that students spend eight to 12 weeks on services in medicine, surgery, pediatrics, obstetrics and gynecology, and psychiatry. Some schools add family practice, while some add other subspecialties. As class sizes grow, schools have had to use increasingly diverse clinical resources to accommodate the students. The result is that quality control is difficult and what is learned varies widely. Even developing a system to really evaluate what should be learned in the clerkship is very difficult. One of my colleagues has conducted studies by direct observation of the clerkships at the University of Illinois. He states that the clerkship is an idiosyncratic learning experience, and that no two students really have the same experience. Another factor which has changed clerkships is that teaching clinical services now are complex, highly technologically based services. It is hard to teach the fundamental skills — such as interviewing and examining patients with simple instruments — when patients are receiving complex diagnostic and therapeutic procedures.

Students' Perceptions of Medical Education

Since 1978, the Association of American Medical Colleges has surveyed students to learn their perceptions of their medical education and what they see as their future plans. A graduation questionnaire is sent to students in December of their senior year, and it is returned some time between December and March. Our response rate has rather consistently been 70 percent; in 1982, 10,938 questionnaires were returned.

As I have mentioned, the fourth year in most schools now is fully elective. Students spend their entire fourth year in clerkships, which are usually a month or six weeks in length, and are of their own choosing. If you look at the elective clerkships that students choose, it's quite clear that the majority feel that they must master the basic technology related to lifesaving measures and radiology. Only three clerkships are reported to have been taken by more than 50 percent of students. Sixty-two percent took a cardiology clerkship, 64 percent took a radiology clerkship, and 53 percent took a clerkship in emergency medicine. I interpret the selection of these clerkships as "getting ready for your internship." In addition, many students use the clerkships to seek a position for their first graduate year. They attempt to take elective clerkships in institutions where they hope to be residents so that they can see and be seen. Forty-seven percent of students responding to the questionnaire last year took elective clerkships in other institutions.

One other area examined in the graduation questionnaire is the views of students regarding emphasis on various areas of medical education. In 1982, 62 percent of the students declared that they had inadequate education in preventive care. When asked about the management of socioeconomic and emotional problems of patients, 47 percent of students said that their experience had been inadequate. Thirty-six percent felt that their experience in the care of ambulatory patients was inadequate. However, 11 percent felt that they had been given inadequate training and experience in interviewing skills. Four percent felt that their hospitalized patient care experience was inadequate, while 96 percent felt that it was either adequate or excessive.

I have painted a rather bleak view of the status of medical education today. Such education is intense; it requires enormous time; and few opportunities are provided for students to be contemplative or to develop process skills. Because of these findings, the Association has embarked on a project which will continue until 1984. Called the General Professional Education of the Physician and College Preparation for Medicine Project, it is supported by the Kaiser Foundation. The project's advisory panel, which consists of 18 members (nine from colleges and universities), is chaired by the President of Johns Hopkins University and co-chaired by the President of the University of Washington. Next I would like to present the panel's concerns.

Concerns and Recommendations of the Project's Panel

There is a broad concensus among panel members that the rate of growth of biomedical knowledge and its application to medical care will increase. The growth and differentiation of knowledge have already caused scientists and physicians to specialize, to pursue knowledge in depth, and to apply it more effectively; the panel believes that this trend will continue. All physicians must be prepared to keep pace with advancing knowledge, and to apply advances that were unforeseen when they were students. To do this requires that students develop the skills, values, and attitudes of learned men and women so that they will continue to learn throughout their professional careers. The panel believes that both college and medical school faculties are currently overwhelming students with details, and that this prevents the development of the scholarly skills and attitudes necessary for continued learning. Great effort must be made to differentiate what must be learned at each stage of medical education. Differentiation should cause the reduction of the degree of detail that students are expected to learn initially and should provide an educational milieu that teaches and reinforces scholarship and independent learning.

Another concern of the panel is the ascendancy of technology. Technical developments have paralleled the growth of knowledge. The application of these inventions to the care of patients has vastly increased the ability of physicians to make diagnoses and treat diseases on the basis of cellular, subcellular, and even molecular abnormalities and dysfunctions. Their introduction has also enhanced the motivation to specialize. The panel is therefore concerned that in the future, physicians may predominantly function as highly skilled, narrowly specialized technologists, who are unable or unwilling to deal with the psychosocial problems of their patients. Because of this concern, the panel believes that all students must learn to interview and listen to patients, and to examine them using basic instruments. In the process of this learning, students should develop sensitivity for the unique qualities of each human being and should learn that physicians are afforded trust and confidence that goes beyond their technical ability. The panel believes that the basic clinical skills are insufficiently emphasized by faculties during clinical education. Emphasis on specialized knowledge and the application of sophisticated technology detracts from students learning the skills that all physicians should have.

The panel foresees that there is a vast and rapid reorganization of the way medical services are being provided. They are concerned that physicians in the future will be operating in large, organized systems, and that their services will be paid for by a relatively few governmental and private agencies. The panel therefore believes that students must learn to work cost-effectively and with other professionals.

Finally, the panel states it is likely that physicians will even be more challenged in the future than now by the rising expectations of a better informed public for sophisticated medical care. They will have to keep abreast of advancing knowledge, practice with externally imposed constraints, and make ethical judgments that will be subjected to critical review. All these challenges will require that physicians acquire healthy modes of coping with stress. Faculties must be sensitive to signs of distress in students, and must intervene to help them develop healthy approaches to coping with stress.

DISCUSSION

Bob Chamberlin: Has there been a growth of social sciences in medical schools' and colleges' curricula?

Gus Swanson: To answer your question, there has been growth to a small degree only. The Association's Curriculum Directory, which has been updated annually since 1972, shows approximately a one percent increase in social sciences.

Chuck Lewis: I would like to mention four groups which are attempting to bring about some of the changes you have mentioned. One is the Society for Primary Research, Education, and Primary Care. It represents essentially clinical department primary care internists. It is an organization which has access to the clinical departments. There is also an Association of Teachers of Behavioral Science that has met for many years and is very concerned with the questions that Bob raised. The third group I would mention is an interesting organization called Human Dimensions in Medical Education, which is in La Jolla, California, at the Institute for the Study of the Person. This group has a sort of "traveling road show" that goes to various medical schools and holds retreats for the faculty to sensitize them to all the issues that we have talked about. It is the only group that I know of that goes into a university and takes away 10 to

15 faculty members and does try to sensitize them and make them aware of the human environment in medical education. The last group is the Institute of Medicine of the National Academy of Science. The Institute is conducting a study of medical education this year. The group's goals are rather enormous in terms of wanting to make curricular changes.

Gus Swanson: My firm belief is that the only way you can change any educational program is to inject an element of doubt in the faculty's mind that what they are doing is absolutely right. In February of 1982, the Association distributed 7,000 copies of a book called *An Overview of the General Professional Education of the Physician;* it raised some questions that we thought should be asked, and brought a fair amount of response from faculties. Another booklet, called *Charges to Working Groups on the Essential Knowledge, Fundamental Skills and Personal Qualities, Values and Attitudes,* has recently been sent to medical schools and to academic societies in teaching hospitals. This document has a number of assumptions and some fairly provocative questions in it. We have invited the medical schools and the societies composed of departmental chairmen to organize discussion groups around it. These efforts are designed to inject an element of doubt among the faculties that what they are doing is absolutely the right thing.

Mary Ann Lewis: I would like to mention that there is a reason that faculty members today do not nurture medical students as they did 20 years ago, and that is that one does not get promoted for teaching medical students. One gets promoted by producing publications that intrigue peers and colleagues. And this is true for all professional students, not just medical students.

Bill Frankenburg: I think the question one might ask is whether the Association agrees with what Mary Ann is saying. And if it does, wouldn't it be appropriate for it to say something to the effect that there ought to be more reward for people in teaching? There really is a universal problem in that we are perpetuating the way we are doing things. People in power in the medical institutions are the ones who have gotten there because of their publications and their research, and that is the way they are going to keep things because that is the most important thing for them.

Gus Swanson: I think one of the outcomes of the Association's whole effort eventually will be a statement along the lines you suggest. Let me point out something I firmly believe in, and that is that the Association of American Medical Colleges does not and should not have autocratic authority over the faculties in this country. We have to convince them to change; we cannot tell them.

Evan Charney: About a decade ago, departments of family medicine became advocates within the medical education system for promoting communication and a psychosocial emphasis in curricula. Frankly, I have given up trying to change the emphasis in pediatrics and internal medicine. In my experience, none of the specialties have ever advocated for this change with more than half a heart because they are caught up in the enormous knowledge explosion you mentioned. This explosion is a reality that those who teach live with every day. The only ones who find psychosocial issues meaningful and important in daily practice are those in primary care disciplines. My hope was that family medicine would strongly advocate for psychosocial curricula emphasis. To what degree has that happened?

Gus Swanson: I have seen materials coming out of the Society for Teachers of Family Medicine to work with local programs to improve quality. The Society really is putting a major emphasis on those areas that concern us. However, the effect on each individual institution is variable and depends upon the locus of the family practice program. In some institutions, family practice has been given a geographic location which ensures that the eyes of a professor of medicine need never fall on the chairman of family practice's door. In other institutions it is different.

It is my private belief that we may be at a point where a paradigm shift is going to come about. The impossibility of continuing to try to teach medical students in depth about everything during four years will become apparent, and there will be an effort to prepare students to learn in depth beyond their undergraduate years.

NURSING EDUCATION

Joy Hinson Penticuff, R.N., Ph.D.

Throughout this Round Table, we have seen the need for improvement in communication between health care providers and children and families. I am pleased to represent the American Association of Colleges of Nursing in presenting an overview of the strengths and weaknesses of nursing curricula, and to give recommendations for improvements in nursing education.

There are currently 284 accredited baccalaureate nursing programs in the United States. To determine how communication is being taught, my staff and I conducted a survey of 23 randomly selected baccalaureate nursing programs in July and August of 1982. Table 1 lists these schools. In addition, we conducted a content analysis of the major undergraduate pediatric nursing textbooks. Information from these two efforts allows me to describe in some detail the most usual curriculum models, pediatric clinical experiences, and pediatric content taught today in American schools of nursing.

Table 1. List of Nursing Schools Surveyed

California State University at Long Beach
Long Beach, California

Loma Linda University
Loma Linda, California

San Diego State University
San Diego, California

San Jose State University
San Jose, California

Valdosta State College
Valdosta, Georgia

Elmhurst College
Elmhurst, Illinois

University of Maryland
Baltimore, Maryland

University of Michigan
Ann Arbor, Michigan

Delta State University
Cleveland, Mississippi

University of Missouri at Columbia
Columbia, Missouri

Montana State University at Bozeman
Bozeman, Montana

Creighton University
Omaha, Nebraska

Union College
Lincoln, Nebraska

College of New Rochelle
New Rochelle, New York

Kent State University
Kent, Ohio

Medical University of South Carolina
Charleston, South Carolina

Tennessee Tech University
Cookeville, Tennessee

Baylor University
Dallas, Texas

University of Texas at Arlington
Arlington, Texas

University of Texas at Austin
Austin, Texas

University of Utah
Salt Lake City, Utah

Radford University
Radford, Virginia

University of Wisconsin at Milwaukee
Milwaukee, Wisconsin

Today, as students begin their first nursing courses, they are exposed to the philosophy that the essence of nursing is the capacity to empathize with others and to be of help. In addition, the students are presented with a strong emphasis on a holistic view of man, with a focus on interpersonal relationships. There is a view of the family rather than the isolated child, and on the influences exerted by the community and environment. Nursing students today are concerned not only with the pathophysiology of illness, but also with how the child and the family adapt to stress produced by illness. Students are increasingly aware that nurses' roles are changing in response to the more informed and active participation of children and families in their own health management. As the nurse-child-family relationship changes, so will the communication process. Judy Igoe's paper has pointed out that it is no longer possible for nurses to remain in the traditional role of authoritarian information-giver, a point with which I agree. We must prepare students so that they will be able to enter into a partnership with families and children for the improvement of health and the prevention of illness.

The results of our survey demonstrate that nursing education emphasizes several conceptual frameworks, as can be seen in Table 2.

Table. 2. Prevalent Conceptual Framework in Nursing Baccalaureate Programs

"Adaptation"
— Interaction between man and environment
— Holistic man
— Maintenance of homeostasis
— Utilization of coping behaviors

"Developmental"
— Human growth and development
— Ages and stages in biological, sociological, psychological, and cognitive domains
— Life cycles from conception to death

"Systems"
— System functioning as a whole through the interdependence of its parts
— Significant terms: boundary, stress, equilibrium, feedback, open system, closed system, subsystem, energy exchange

Note—Santora, D. Conceptual frameworks used in baccalaureate and master's degree curricula. Publication No. 15-1828, New York: National League for Nursing, 1980.

Foremost are theories of crisis and adaptation, of development and growth, of change as part of life; in addition, emphasis is placed on concepts relating to the complexities of interpersonal relationships and human behavior. Table 3 illustrates Infante's crisis theory framework.

The reason for including Infante's framework is for the purpose of illustrating how complex nursing theory has become. The conceptual

Table 3.

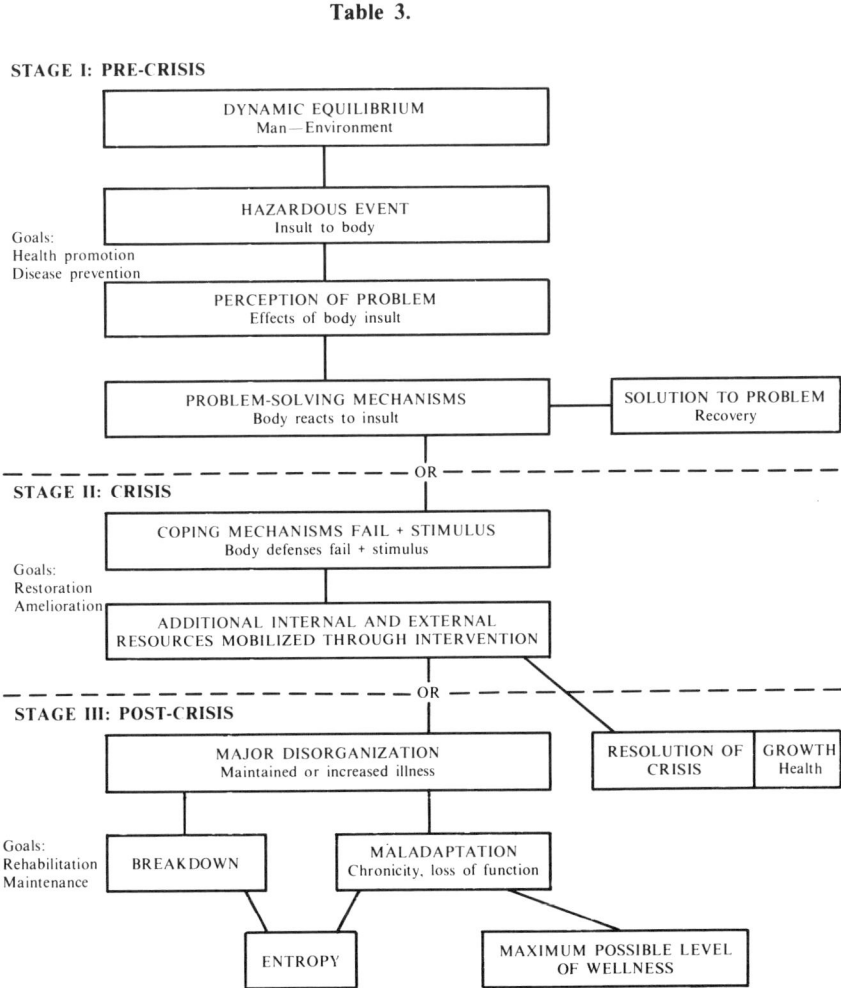

Prepared by the faculty of The University of Connecticut School of Nursing

Note:—Mary Sue Infante, editor *Crisis Theory: A Framework for Nursing Practice.* Pg. 14 Reprinted with permission of Reston Publishing Co., Inc. A Prentice-Hall Company, 11480 Sunset Hills Road, Reston, Virginia 22090.

framework given in Table 3 is currently being used in baccalaureate nursing programs, and indeed such complex frameworks are usual in the majority of baccalaureate nursing programs today. Such humanistic ideals are a part of nursing values. Yet these views of man and of the nurse's role in assisting man surely create expectations that these ideals will be put into nursing practice. The students expect that, upon graduation, they will be able to put into practice the philosophical and conceptual frameworks which underlie our basic nursing curricula today.

Description of Typical Baccalaureate Program

Table 4 describes a typical baccalaureate nursing program. Students enter most baccalaureate nursing programs after two years of

Table 4. Structure of a Typical Baccalaureate Nursing Program

Freshman and Sophomore Years

Pre-Nursing Requisite Courses
Psychology, Child Development

Junior Year

Foundational Nursing Concepts and Processes
— Philosophy of nursing
— Holistic man
— Self-concept
— Mental health concepts
— Nursing within interpersonal relationships
— Principles of communication (verbal/nonverbal, congruence, empathy)
— "Helping relationships"
— Initial contact with well, ambulatory preschoolers
— Movement from well individuals to ill families

Senior Year

Specialized Clinical Nursing Courses
— Pediatric nursing
— High-risk perinatal nursing
— The chronically disabled child
— Movement from family illness to community problems and methods for primary intervention

Note—American Association of Colleges of Nursing Survey Data, 1982.

nursing prerequisite courses, which include introductory psychology and child development. Initial nursing courses focus on the holistic nature of man, basic interviewing skills, verbal and nonverbal communication, and the development of what is termed the "helping relationship."

In most colleges of nursing, students are exposed to commercially and faculty prepared videotapes describing appropriate communication in situations portraying adults. Yet our survey indicates that relatively few programs (16 percent) videotape students interacting with families. Pittman at Florida State University, and Farrell and others at Worcester State College have published details of their semester-long interpersonal skills courses which could serve as models for nursing schools wishing to employ videotape techniques. I recommend that nursing programs use these technologies to develop clinical evaluation instruments, and to give students feedback about their interaction with families and children.

Our survey demonstrates that initial student contact with young children is generally focused on physical and developmental assessment of the child. Students have only very brief contact at this time with the families of children.

As can be seen from Table 4, an elective pediatric rotation is offered during the student's senior year in a typical school of nursing. There are usually pediatric placements — most of them in acute care settings — available for about one-third of the student body. Our survey indicates that nursing instructors spend the majority of their clinical time teaching procedures and technical skills rather than in focusing on supervision of student-child-family interaction. Indeed, we found that most instructors spend only an average of five to 10 percent of clinical time in direct supervision of student-family or student-child interaction.

We also inquired about the methods instructors use to evaluate a student's communication, and what proportion of the student's grade is based on communication skills. Approximately seven percent of the schools reported that they use a structured, objective tool to evaluate student communication within the clinical laboratory. In most programs, grading is on a pass/fail basis, with the instructor making a subjective judgment as to how well the student has mastered communication skills.

The amount of student interaction with families of institutionalized children varies. Children of poverty-level families may not have access to lodging near some referral hospitals. Another important factor has to do with the amount of time the hospitalized child's family is allowed to remain with the child. A study of Fagin and Nusbaum revealed that only 62 percent of hospital pediatric services in the United States allowed unlimited visiting for parents. In addition, in those hospitals with 24-hour rooming-in, no more than 20 percent of parents were with their children at the time of the study. While there is much support for the idea of parent involvement in the care of the child and the need for families to plan a treatment regimen which they can carry out, it seems that nursing education has thus far failed to have a significant influence in hospital practice settings. Restrictions on family visitation continue to be in effect in some areas in spite of convincing evidence (by Fagin and Nusbaum) of the risks to young children of separation during illness.

Thus another of my recommendations is that parents and consumers organize and conduct periodic policy review of all pediatric institutions. This would help ensure that the structure of nursing practice is consistent with the needs and goals of children and families, and it would allow nurses to participate in consumer-designed and consumer-evaluated pediatric services.

Most students do work closely with families, but less often with families in crisis. Our survey showed that undergraduate pediatric instructors usually do not assign students to work with families and children in acute crisis situations. However, Dunlop at Boston College has implemented a course in crisis intervention as an elective in the basic nursing education program which might serve as a model for other nursing schools.

In most acute-care pediatric placements, students are introduced to play interviews and play as a therapeutic activity. It is usually only at the graduate level, however, that students begin to study the uses and interpretation of play with sick children in depth.

Content Analysis of Pediatric Textbooks

The content relevant to communication with children and families as presented in those textbooks (Table 5) used in the majority of undergraduate pediatric nursing courses was analyzed. The universal content found is presented in Table 6. As can be seen, issues such as separation and loss, control and competence, mobility, activity, and isolation — as these are affected by illness — are presented in all the nursing programs studied. In addition, illness is described as a situation which has the potential outcome for the child and family of either crisis or growth. The meaning of illness from the child's viewpoint and developmental changes in children's views of illness causality are universally presented, as is the meaning of illness to family members and family reactions to illness and hospitalization. Another area commonly presented has to do with developmental changes in children's ability to cope with illness and hospital experiences, as well as the impact of illness and hospitalization on cognitive, emotional, and social behavior. Nursing care to promote growth and constructive coping during the various developmental phases of childhood, concentrating on the involvement of the family in both planning and caretaking of the child, are also presented in all the textbooks surveyed.

Table 5. Prevalent Undergraduate Pediatric Textbooks Submitted to Communication Content Analysis

Marlow, D.R. *Textbook of pediatric nursing* (5th ed.). Philadelphia, PA: W.B. Saunders Company, 1977.

Pillitteri, A. *Nursing care of the growing family: A child health text.* Boston, MA: Brown and Company, 1977.

Scipien, G.M., Barnard, M.U., Chard, M.A., Howe, J. & Phillips, P.J. *Comprehensive pediatric nursing.* New York: McGraw-Hill Book Company, 1979.

Tackett, J.J.M. & Hunsberger, M. *Family centered care of children and adolescents: Nursing concepts in child health.* Philadelphia, PA: J.B. Lippincott Company, 1976.

Waley, L.F. & Wong, D.L. *Nursing care of infants and children.* St. Louis, MO: The C.V. Mosby Company, 1979.

Our content analysis revealed not only what students are being taught today, but also revealed gaps in essential content. For example, as Eland has noted, the textbooks deal inadequately with the significance of children's acute and chronic pain. Another area that is inadequately covered is the institutional abuse of children.

Communication Within the Context of Helping Relationships

The challenge to nursing education is to prepare professional nurses who are sensitive to psychosocial needs and capable of helping children and families cope more effectively with stress. Our survey results indicate that, upon completion of their baccalaureate degree, nursing students who have taken specialized undergraduate courses in pediatrics (approximately one-third of the students) are very aware of the stresses that families and children are under when children are ill. They do view families and children in terms of the entirety of human functioning, they are aware of the significance of relation-

Table 6. Content Universally Presented in Texts

Separation and loss
Control and competence
Mobility
Activity
Isolation
Illness as crisis or growth potential
Meaning of illness to children of different ages
Meaning of illness to families
Child's reactions to illness/hospitalization
Family's reactions to illness/hospitalization
Coping with illness/treatment: Developmental issues
Illness impact on cognitive, emotional, social behavior
Involvement of child and family in planning and care

---

ships, and they can distinguish between supportive and troubled relationships. Yet it is possible that this very awareness of the humanness of children and families, and the students' insights into their own humanity, may leave them vulnerable to disappointment within the practice setting after graduation. The complexity of our current nursing philosophical and scientific viewpoints provides the widest possible scope in our attempts to understand human behavior and to nurture human coping and growth. But this evolving understanding has been only incompletely translated into nursing practice.

Nurses have long held the notion that they should be all things to all people. The fact is, the practice of nursing is stressful, and the practice of pediatric nursing is especially so. I recommend the facilitation of stronger support systems for nurses within the agencies where they work, with formal opportunities for planning and evaluating child health care communication. Crisis intervention for nurses may be an appropriate role for a master's-prepared mental health nurse clinician. At the same time, each nurse needs to develop both a personal and a professional support system, or, as Gortner phrases it, "strategies for survival in the practice world."

Students are supervised in clinical lab during nursing education, and when they are confronted with difficult issues — such as ethical dilemmas, child malnutrition, abuse, and neglect, and decisions about professional integrity — they are encouraged to participate in value clarification and ethical debate. These progressive mechanisms need to be instituted in pediatric health care settings as well.

The implementation of primary nursing — in which one nurse has an ongoing, central relationship with the child and family — is a structure which allows the development of relationships over time. The opportunity to get to know the child and family more closely and to be responsible for the nursing care given has the effect of increasing nurses' sense of being able to "make a difference" in the ultimate outcome for the child and family.

The Need for Collaboration between Nurse Educators and Nurse Clinicians

I have made a number of recommendations in the course of this presentation, and these are summarized in Table 7. One final overall recommendation is for increased collaboration between nurse educators and nurses in full-time clinical practice, a strategy which would have a number of positive outcomes. Such collaboration could include dual appointments, collaborative clinical research, and use of staff preceptors as expert role models.

Collaboration between educational and practice institutions would allow faculty members to engage in clinical practice and thereby be the necessary models of expert interaction with children and families. Dual appointments (of nursing faculty to clinical positions in pediatric agencies, and appointment of clinical staff to lectureship positions) would facilitate faculty practice and decrease clinical staff burnout. Teaching and research positions for clinical staff can help to put the stressful realities of practice into a more balanced perspective, thereby enhancing the staff's ability for self-renewal and leading them

---

Table 7. Summary of Recommendations

Recognition of experiential nature of learning how to communicate

Formal collaboration between academic and practice institutions

Use of expert role models in complex practice situations

Periodic institutional policy reviews

Implementation of primary nursing

Support systems in the practice setting

Preventive mental health specialists within the practice settings: Role funding, development, and research

Clinical nursing research on how to improve child health care communications

to be more available to care for children and families in distress.

DISCUSSION

Mary Ann Lewis: I think the technology that is affecting medical education is also affecting nursing education. The difference is that nursing education does not have any significant training relationships with hospitals. I think that the so-called nursing shortage that we are having in hospitals today is the result. Hospitals are very rigid, hierarchical, bureaucratic organizations that have not changed since the Dark Ages. And until those structures are willing to be more flexible, and to allow the professional practice of nursing, I think nurses are going to continue to avoid practicing in hospitals.

Suzie Rimstidt: Joy, I want to endorse the primary nursing concept, both in the hospital and out. I am pleased to see that primary nursing is being instituted in many progressive hospitals in the country. The problem I see is that primary nursing takes its toll on nurses, because they become more intimate and involved with families. I think this is a good pattern, but nurses need to be emotionally supported as they move into more patient involvement.

Lee Schorr: It seems to me that we are getting back to the issue of who should be the primary communicator with families. I saw an incident which I think is relevant here and which I would like to share. I sat in on rounds in a children's hospital where one of the cases that was being discussed was that of a 14-year-old girl with cystic fibrosis. All the physicians on the house staff who had contact with the girl were persuaded that this was her terminal hospitalization. They speculated about what the girl knew about her condition, what the attending physician knew, and about who had communicated with whom on that subject. Everybody in the room knew that nobody there knew, and they also all knew that the nurses knew. The most striking thing to me was how content they were to leave communication to the nurses, and how they felt that perhaps the nurses would talk to the attending physician and to the family. On the one hand, I felt good that the physicians were so confident that the nurses were taking care of all communication. On the other hand, I thought the nurses should be on the rounds so that the physicians would know what was happening.

Joy Penticuff: The point, it seems to me, is that having sensitive, communicative nurses is only going to be optimally effective if there is a connection between what they do and what the physicians are doing.

Lorna Facteau: Perhaps the medical model of the internship might be one way of decreasing burnout that occurs in hospitals, and of decreasing culture shock. Perhaps it would also improve the product.

Joy Penticuff: I agree. It is our responsibility to prepare nurses to function in the real world of the hospital. I feel that we have had our heads in the sand to a certain extent for a number of years, and that we must prepare nurses not only to survive in hospitals, but to grab some power from the institutions and make important changes in them.

Evan Charney: I think Joy has identified an interesting point, which is that nursing educators have done a better job than medical educators in giving students the kind of psychosocial curriculum that this Round Table has been talking about. But nursing educators have not prepared their students for the real world, where they will work, so some of that information is useless. I want to make one advertisement here, if you will. I think that nurses have abandoned community hospitals inappropriately; they have run to the university hospitals so they could have degrees. Yet two-thirds of the children in this country are cared for at community hospitals, and they need effective, caring nurses.

Joy Penticuff: Evan, while I recognize the difficulty some community hospitals have in staffing their facility with nurses, I do not think it is accurate to conclude that nurses have "run to the university hospitals so they could have degrees." Nurses today are committed to excellence in practice, which motivates many of them to seek postgraduate nursing degrees in specialty areas, it is true. But there are other reasons that community hospitals have trouble getting and keeping nurses. Many of them are not as progressive in dealing with children and their families as university hospitals, which poses a problem for nurses who are trained to deal with the patient as a whole person. Many community hospitals do not offer the same level of sophisticated care as university hospitals, which means that nurses with specialty degrees cannot make full use of their skills. I think that nurses and others involved with community hospitals need to work to make those hospitals more caring and more involved with the whole child and family. Then perhaps community hospitals will have less trouble attracting nurses.

PRACTICING NURSE PRACTITIONERS

Karen Fond, R.N., M.S.N.

The expanded role of nursing, as exemplified by nurse practitioners (NPs), was born in the late 1960s because of a perceived shortage of primary care providers. Today, the National Board of Pediatric Nurse Practitioners/Associates estimates that 5,500 pediatric nurse practitioners (PNPs) have graduated from recognized programs, and some 200 more students are expected to graduate each year. The majority will hold a master's level degree, and increasing numbers of PNPs will work in community-based facilities, and hospitals' ambulatory and inpatient units. While nurses historically worked directly with patients, indirect services such as administrative duties, case coordination, and patient management have increasingly pulled nurses away from personal contact. The nurse practitioner model has restored involvement with patients and has changed the direction of nursing in a positive and probably permanent way.

Educating Nurse Practitioners for Communication

Early NP educational programs did not focus heavily on communication in an erroneous assumption that, because students were graduate nurses with clinical experience, they could effectively interview, counsel, and educate patients. Yet studies showed that this was not true, so course material was changed. Today, most NP programs include three required quarter or semester courses designed to examine theories of individual and family dynamics, with a major focus on interpersonal behavior patterns. Didactic material is integrated with real or simulated clinical situations so that students can apply the principles they have learned. Skills are taught in sequential steps beginning with simple observation and listening, moving to role playing of complex problems, and resulting in actual work with clinically stressed patients. Techniques commonly used are videotapes, audiotapes, process recordings, small group role playing and discussion, case presentations, clinical preceptorships, and self-prescriptions and evaluations.

PNPs, who will assume whole visit responsibility and be identified with pediatricians, must also be aware of and sensitive to factors which influence doctor-patient communications. Certain key references are used by PNP faculty members, of which the most well known are those by Korsch et al. Her writing directs students to listen to parents' major worries, ask about their expectations, demonstrate warmth, take time for questions and explanations, explain treatment plans in terms of worries and expectations, and offer availability and support. For example, parents of a sick child need to understand the diagnosis and the nature and cause of the illness before they are satisfied. Parents often feel guilty, fearing that they caused an illness or didn't recognize symptoms quickly enough; thus a clear statement of the child's condition, of its cause and expected course, and of helpful treatment plans alleviates parental anxiety.

A number of researchers have shown that parents have difficulty voicing their concerns and expectations. During post-visit interviews, Korsch, Gozzi, and Francis found that 24 percent of parents' main worries and 65 percent of their expectations were not verbalized to the doctor. Although the pediatricians involved believed that they had allowed ample opportunity for questions, 10 percent of the mothers asked no questions at all, and 27 percent asked only one or two. Bain has also documented this communication gap with family physicians where, in 24 percent of the visits studied, parents asked no questions and, in 51 percent of the visits, no verbal responses were made to physician instructions. Bain has postulated that when the provider controls the consultation, an authoritarian status is created which can intimidate patients. Counseling — in the form of advice — often also falls victim to this trap when the patient is confronted with a problem identified by the advisor who then proceeds to outline ideas on what the patient should do to change. This can make the patient feel inferior and foolish, and can create feelings of inadequacy and helplessness. Collins reminds practitioners that effective communication is not a natural consequence of the helping commitment. She emphasizes the need for mutual patient-professional problem-solving and decision-making. She proposes changing the focus from nurse-patient to patient-nurse, which returns the control to the patient — its rightful owner.

Practice with Individual Children

Given that NPs begin practice prepared with some knowledge, awareness, and experience in effective communication, what are

PNPs doing to improve child health care? It is my pleasure to share a few articles on PNPs' work with children, parent groups, and mothers as selected examples, and to comment on what more can be done in the future.

As PNPs, we are concerned about children and how to effectively relate to them. Because a good portion of communication is language-based and verbally oriented, we must adapt approaches to children's developmental capabilities. We know that cognitive ability to understand words as symbols as well as proficiency in speaking develop over time, so with young children PNPs can focus on such nonverbal modes as behavior cues.

Moss has described signs of cooperation exhibited by two- to four-year-olds during physical examination, which is a potentially threatening experience. The child who makes eye contact, reaches for an offered toy, and is willing to talk with the examiner is signaling a readiness to be approached or even touched. The PNP who makes portions of the developmental and neurological examination into games helps the child gain a sense of comfort and mastery over the situation. Giving choices as to location of the examination (mother's lap or table) as well as the next body part to be examined also communicates to children that they are partners in this health venture. Thus the quality of the interaction between the nurse and child transcends the mere gathering of information. Cooperative behavior during the physical examination is a desirable occurrence for the practitioner, parent, and child, of course, but of more significance is the fact that nurses who watch for behavioral signals from children can actively involve and invest children in their own health care.

Children's artwork has also been studied extensively as a means of discovering children's feelings. Examining a child's art is another nonverbal modality which nurses and other professionals can use to see how children are coping with stresses encountered in the health facility. Allen has described her work in preparing children for hospitalization by looking at their pictures. She found that when six- to 12-year-olds were initially asked to draw what it would be like to be in the hospital, their portraits were fearful, faulty, and confused. They drew bars on windows and beds, small child figures in relationship to doctors and nurses, enormous instruments which inflicted pain floating in the air, and a predominance of red and black colors representing blood, hurt, and death. After a teaching session about hospitalization which included active play with hospital equipment, subsequent pictures contained more appropriately sized people and instruments, smiling faces, and an increase in happy green, yellow, and blue colors.

Those experienced with interpreting children's art agree that the size and detail in which a figure is drawn indicates its importance to the child. Objects of personal or repeated experience, or those having special emotional meaning, are likely to be larger and more detailed than others. The use of red and black colors as symbolic of hurt and death are also recognized from as early as four years. As Allen has shown, the effectiveness of a teaching intervention can be evaluated in terms of changes in children's art; this technique can also be used in other situations such as preparing children to visit the dentist, go to school, have a sibling, and so on.

To learn whether teaching can affect not only knowledge but also attitudes and behaviors, Adams studied the effects of an educational program about seat belt use in cars. Pre-tests given to both experimental and control groups of fifth graders did not differ significantly. However, the experimental group scored substantially higher in knowledge items on the post-test, while the control group showed no change. Attitudinally, no change occurred in either group in their basic like or dislike of seat belts, but of those children who liked the belts, 45 percent reported wearing one during their last ride whereas only six percent who disliked the belts wore one. (Of interest is the fact that only 15 percent of parent drivers wore seat belts, but there was a significant positive relationship between parents and child both using belts.) On pre- and post-testing, 72 percent of the sample reported not wearing belts, thus leading to the conclusion that giving children information alone does not promote belt usage or change attitudes, and that parental role modeling is a significant factor. (Reasons the children gave for disliking and not using seat belts were that they were difficult to reach, were hard to fasten and unfasten, were hot, and were the cause of a feeling of pain at the neck and around the waist. These can be useful directives to change the characteristics of seat belts before expecting children to use them.)

Practice with Parent Groups

In the spirit of teamwork, patients and professionals alike have stimulated the formation of groups as a method of purposefully communicating about and coping with particular health issues. Within the group, the professional has a definite role, usually as leader and/or facilitator. Lay members usually provide mutual emotional support, and share personal experiences and knowledge which can help all members — including the professional — solve problems.

Parents of chronically ill or disabled children have especially benefited from participation in groups. Through the groups they gain better understanding of their child's condition and improve their ability to meet everyday, lifelong stresses. A particularly effective group, the Parents of Asthmatic Kids, has been reported by Walsh, a PNP who helped form it. Parents who became involved wanted medical information on asthma, medications, nutrition, physical activity, breathing exercises, and relaxation techniques; they also wanted to explore their feelings about having an asthmatic child and such issues as the effects of asthma on family relationships, school problems, management of summer vacations, behavior modification. The asthmatic children were included in a separate group, where cartoons and videotapes on asthma, breathing games, and vital capacity challenges were viewed as fun. An exciting spinoff that might only have evolved from group identification was the formation of a siblings' group to help brothers and sisters also understand asthma and to explore their feelings of resentment and frustration. The positive results of this group were a dramatic decrease in acute office visits as well as an increase in parental feelings of competency and satisfaction. Thus, Walsh has written that a "parent support group can be an inexpensive, efficient and rewarding way to educate a family and its children about an illness and its management."

Practice with Mothers

As this Round Table has emphasized, eliciting the perceptions of parents is necessary in a whole communication effort. Of the many strategies developed to elicit parents' perceptions, the simplest can often be most revealing. One approach used at UCLA to identify mothers' expectations in communicating with pediatricians was to invite a panel of mothers into the classroom to meet with pediatric residents. This forum was less threatening than individual sessions in answering the question of what mothers want from their pediatricians.

In general, the mothers who met with the residents said that they often felt looked down upon by the doctor, and that they wished to be viewed as having a valuable opinion and as being capable of making a good decision. Professional women, especially, felt competent in their work but less so in their mothering role. The mothers said that the physician's phrase, "Don't worry," is deadly. They noted that if they voiced a complaint to the physician, they felt either something was wrong with the baby or that they themselves needed attention from the doctor. Mothers readily admit that they talk with other parents to find a satisfactory pediatrician who really listens to their concerns.

All mothers who telephone the physician with a problem want to have their calls returned. They find it hard to repeatedly impose on doctors, perceiving that physicians are extremely busy, and are afraid to say that their situation is an emergency. Mothers also want their pediatrician to like children, and want time from the physician after a long wait. As Korsch found, mothers expect the physician to be friendly, concerned, and sympathetic, and to take time for questions and explanations.

PNPs need to know what mothers expect from them in comparison to physicians, since there are differences in knowledge base and scope and depth of medical practice that might define differences in communication and relationship. Do mothers bring up different subjects with PNPs? Do they find PNPs more approachable, as reflected by asking many more questions? Do they seek emergency room care with physicians when they perceive their children to be very ill rather than call their PNP? The early NP studies focused on topics related to the nurse's new role, such as delegation of medical functions, adequacy of care provided, acceptance by physicians, and patient satisfaction. Thus the literature for 10 years was devoted to descriptions of various roles and settings where NPs were effective providers. Only in the last five years have studies been conducted into nurse-parent/child interactions. These studies have recognized that more emphasis into communication variables is needed. For example, recent research has investigated the effects of childbirth education on parent-infant relationships, the effectiveness of audiovisual aids in promoting parenting skills for teen-agers, the effects of catheterization on attitudes of myelodysplastic children, and parents' perceived needs in child health clinics.

Other Areas of Practice: Teaching and Research

PNPs also affect child health care through teaching and research. University-based PNPs precept NP, medical, and dental students, teaching them elements of developmental assessment, nutritional counseling, health maintenance, interviewing and history-taking, and so on.

PNPs in specialty areas teach a wide range of other people. For example, the Neurology PNP at Children's Hospital of Los Angeles teaches school teachers, school nurses, and children with seizure disorders about seizures and medication. This same PNP coordinates the home evaluation and family functioning activities of public health nurses. Some PNPs also lecture formally to professionals at grand rounds, morning case conferences, and housestaff care series, while some make presentations to consumer and school groups.

Another area in which PNPs contribute to child health care is research. PNPs have focused on research into the nonverbal communication of children, and into communication via children's artwork. The results of these PNP research efforts have been described earlier in this presentation.

In summary, improvement of pediatric care through improved communication is a goal of practitioners in both nursing and medicine. Any advancement toward this goal will be dependent initially upon the quality of teaching (including both theoretical knowledge and clinical practicums) provided in organized educational programs. Practicing health professionals have a responsibility to recognize problems deriving from faulty interpersonal communication with children, parents, and families, and to develop some strategies leading to successful resolutions. Those who can will study interaction variables in more organized and empirical paradigms, thus tackling the subjective and interpretive difficulty of communication.

What is clear, as this Round Table attests, is that the results of all our efforts must be reported so that what is known will be constantly expanded and refined. The NP field is in its infancy in generating new information relating to communication in pediatric care, but as it progresses with more studies like those reported, exciting findings are expected from PNPs in the future.

DISCUSSION

Mary Ann Lewis: It seems to me that NP models are upgrading nursing skills in general. Perhaps in years to come, this will increase the number of nurses going back into hospitals who will be better prepared with better diagnostic and assessment skills.

Bob Chamberlin: What are the legal restrictions now in terms of the supervision of NPs? Can NPs practice in satellite clinics without a physician actually on site in most states if they are in contact with a physician in another place? Or does a supervising physician have to actually be present?

Karen Fond: It depends upon the state, since nursing practice is defined by individual state's Boards of Nursing. Most often these boards work in collaboration with medical boards, and supervision by a physician is usually specified in broad terms. Often supervision is by telephone, for example, and is not defined in terms of numbers of miles between the NP and the physician. The quality of the relationship is generally left up to the NP and the supervising physician.

Bob Pantell: A number of years ago, I saw that NP programs were training a large number of subspecialists. I am not talking about pediatric generalists, but about such specialists as the pediatric cardiology NPs. I wonder if the same specialization training is still continuing, or if there has been a retrenchment.

Karen Fond: I do think that NPs are continuing to specialize in areas in subspecialty medical practice where there has been a need for continuity of patient care — for coordination or for complex medical management. As I said earlier, as fellowships in medicine decrease, more reliance is put on the NP in specialty areas.

THE PHYSICIAN'S ROLE AS A COMMUNICATOR IN CHILD HEALTH CARE

James E. Strain, M.D.

This conference has focused on the importance of communications in the delivery of health care, on the need to improve health care communications, and on strategies for teaching better communication. I will attempt to discuss the physician's role as a communicator from the perspective of a practicing pediatrician in an ambulatory setting. I would like to first comment on how information is exchanged in a patient visit to a physician; second, discuss the unique aspects of communication in child health care; and third, conclude with suggestions for the education of the physician in techniques of good communication.

Communication During A Health Care Visit

Communication is the essence of good patient care. Without an open exchange of information, thoughts, and ideas between physician and patient, health care becomes stereotyped and mechanical. It is important to remember that good communication involves listening as well as talking. Communication also occurs in subtle, nonverbal ways, and a perceptive physician can use knowledge of nonverbal communication to discern feelings and attitudes that may be extremely important in the care of the patient.

Conceptually, communication occurs between patient and physician in three phases. The first is the history as related by the patient. A visit to the physician is usually initiated by the patient because of a specific concern. The physician must remember that the patient is the most important — and often the only — source of information about his or her illness or health status. Thus obtaining information from the patient is essential in making an accurate diagnosis and meeting the patient's needs. An important measure of patient satisfaction is how well the physician deals with the specific concerns of the patient. Unless the physician is aware of those concerns, it's unlikely that they will be addressed.

The interview usually begins with a question about the presenting complaint. The real reason for the visit may not be apparent at first, but will often be uncovered later in the discussion. The physician may need to ask questions to clarify the details of the present illness, past history, systems review, and family history, but it's important that this not be ritualistic and that the patient be given time to respond to questions in a meaningful way. The patient should not only be encouraged to describe symptoms in his or her own words, but to express feelings, anxieties, and fears as well.

There are barriers to good communication in this phase of the physician visit. The first is a time constraint. Although appointment systems usually allow for flexibility, unexpected delays, emergencies, and special problems that require more time than anticipated often interfere with the orderly conduct of patient care. If time does not permit satisfactory communication between physician and patient, another appointment should be arranged to complete what was started on the first visit.

Another pitfall that the physician must be aware of and avoid is making a diagnosis on the basis of incomplete information. In the course of an interview, the physician may reach a conclusion before the patient has related all the details of the illness. If the history is incomplete, errors will be made in diagnosis.

The second phase of communication between patient and physician follows the physical examination and laboratory studies. The physician must communicate findings and conclusions clearly to the patient, and time must be allowed for questions. Medical terms commonly used by physicians are often misunderstood or not understood at all by patients, so they should be avoided or explained in detail. Patients are sometimes reluctant to admit they don't completely understand the physician's explanation, so discussion of the diagnosis should be invited. It's not uncommon for a patient to "miss" part of the discussion, particularly if the level of anxiety over an illness is high. In stressful situations, important information may bear repeating.

A third phase of communication deals with management and treatment. The key to this important aspect of the visit is the patient's understanding of the reason for a specific treatment. Many patients are knowledgeable about the use of medications, their side effects, and their contraindications (the *Physician's Desk Reference* can be purchased in most book stores). Other patients have only a superficial knowledge of the effects of medication. In either case, a clear explanation should be given for why medications have been ordered, with time allowed for questions. Compliance is directly related to the understanding of the intended outcome of treatment.

In addition, in our litigious society, physicians have become acutely aware of the need to keep patients informed. It's been shown that a good patient-physician relationship reduces the likelihood of malpractice claims, and that the relationship can best be maintained through open and ongoing communication. As in any human endeavor, errors are made in patient management, and treatment results are sometime poor through no fault of the physician. In either case, good communication tends to dispel the misunderstanding, disappointment, and anger that often are the geneses of malpractice suits.

Communication Regarding Child Health

I want to discuss next the unique opportunities for communication in child health care. This may begin before conception, when parents seek genetic advice about a familial disorder.

In other instances, the first communication may take place during a prenatal visit to the physician who will be caring for the child. This visit is now being widely promoted by obstetricians and pediatricians. It is an excellent opportunity for the physician to become acquainted with the parents, to understand their concerns, and to discuss philosophies of child rearing and parenting. Questions can be answered about labor and delivery, the examination and screening tests done in the hospital, and the ongoing care of the child after discharge. The visit gives the physician the opportunity to discuss such matters as breast feeding, circumcision, and the purchase of an infant car seat. Parents can be reassured of the availability of the physician if problems occur during labor or delivery.

In most cases, communication is natural and easy in the postnatal period. Parents are eager to know about the specifics of infant care and are extremely receptive to advice and counsel. This is also an enjoyable experience for the physician, who shares in the family's excitement over the new baby.

The ongoing care of the child after discharge from the newborn nursery usually includes periodic visits to the child's physician. These visits include taking a history and conducting a physical examination; but more importantly, they address the concerns of the parents. In addition, these visits permit the physician to give parents important information and advice about nutrition, infant stimulation, anticipatory guidance, and accident prevention. (Several studies have documented the correlation between repeated communications with parents about infant car seats and the actual use of the seats.) The two-way communication that occurs during health supervision visits gives the parents confidence in their own parenting abilities and fosters a close personal relationship between the physician and the family.

In recent years more fathers have become involved in the care of their children, and often they accompany their wives to the physician's office or clinic. This is a healthy trend that allows the physician to communicate with both parents about their individual concerns. Information given to parents should be clear and concise. At the same time, independent decision-making should be encouraged, for parents need to develop confidence in their own judgment and abilities.

As the child grows older, communication between physician and parents continues to be an important part of child health care, but now the *child* becomes a communicator, and it is important for the physician to recognize him or her as an important source of information. In the case of illnesses, the child can usually give an accurate description of the symptoms. For example, when a child complains of an earache, an ear infection is almost always present. At the time of periodic examinations, counseling about accident prevention should be directed to the child as well as the parents. Behavioral disorders, school failure, and disruptions in the family — including death and divorce — are not uncommon in this age group, and the physician must communicate with the child directly to effectively deal with the problems. The physician can also help parents communicate with their children as the children grow and develop. Books for both parents and children may be recommended to facilitate this communication.

In the care of adolescents, the physician must make a transition from being the physician to the parent to being the physician to the young adult. This transition is sometimes difficult for parents to understand and accept, but a relationship between the adolescent and the physician that ensures confidentiality must be established. Young people often have a closer relationship with their peers than their parents, and an understanding adult can be of enormous help during this important stage of development. The physician who has known a teen-ager from early childhood is often the best person to counsel the adolescent. The psychosocial disorders of adolescence, including developing sexuality, teen-age pregnancy, mental disturbances, and substance abuse require prompt intervention by a caring, understanding adult.

Telephone communication is an important part of child health care. Many problems, including the management of minor illnesses, can be resolved by telephone discussion. Many times this advice is given by an experienced nurse or physician's assistant. It's important for the physician and nurse to communicate freely about management of specific problems so there is consistency and continuity in the information being given. Some physicians prefer to limit telephone communication by making a charge for the service or by limiting the telephone hours; however, in my view the telephone should be an open line of communication, and barriers should not be imposed to limit its use. If parents are unable to reach their physician, they will get their information from other, less reliable sources.

Strategies for Teaching Physicians Communication Skills

How can physicians be educated in the art of communication? Numerous strategies for teaching better communication have been discussed during this meeting. Workshops and round tables are suitable formats and can include videotaping of interviews, role playing, presentations by parents, and case studies that demonstrate the importance of communication in patient care.

Logically, these could be presented as continuing medical education (CME) courses. However, it should be understood that physicians are deluged with promotional material on a wide variety of CME programs, and priority will be given to courses that are most interesting and most practical and useful in the delivery of health care. Therefore, physicians must be convinced that communication skills are important and that knowledge acquired in CME courses will be useful in the care of their patients. Articles in scientific publications, including the specialty journals, may be one way to stimulate physicians' interest. Techniques proposed for improving patient-physician communication must be practical and realistic, and take into account time constraints of practice.

A physician who is an active member of a clinical or volunteer faculty is frequently called upon to instruct students or serve as a preceptor to pediatric residents. A major contribution that faculty members can make to university teaching programs is the demonstration of communication skills. This includes interview techniques, explaining the results of the physical examination and laboratory tests to children and their families, and giving children and their parents understandable instructions about treatment. In demonstrating communication skills, the teacher becomes the learner. Not only does the student benefit from observing the physician, but the physician becomes more aware of his or her own abilities to communicate with patients in a meaningful way.

DISCUSSION

Bob Chamberlin: The latest study of pediatric practice shows that the average pediatrician spends about 90 seconds in anticipatory guidance during each patient visit. What implications do you see for training pediatricians in the way practice is structured?

Jim Strain: I really think pediatricians need more training in ambulatory settings. Currently, we train tertiary care pediatricians. They are very, very good at fluid and electrolyte management, but they need more experience in ambulatory care. I am a proponent of conducting training in a physician's office where an effective role model can have an impact.

Bob Chamberlin: I see structural barriers to training in pediatricians' offices because any primary care practice is essentially a volume practice, and the physician has to see a fair number of patients. In addition, the whole reimbursement mechanism is set up to discourage spending any extra time with patients because physicians do not get reimbursed for it.

Jim Strain: That is right. If a physician has a student or resident in the office, he or she will have to schedule fewer visits. A physician role model has to be able to spend more time with the student and with the family. A physician does pay a price economically to be a mentor to a student. Unfortunately, there is just no way that we are going to be able to pay volunteer or clinical faculty for the time they spend with students. For example, at the University of Colorado last year, 8,000 hours were given by volunteer clinical faculty in training students at all levels. But Colorado's experience does show, I think, that with careful organization and structuring of what happens in the office, we can provide more ambulatory training for medical students and residents.

Lee Schorr: Getting back to the question of the time it takes to communicate, Barbara Korsch found that communication did not take a lot of additional time. Morris Green says it is like juggling, that at first you can only get one ball up at a time, but as you get better and better, you can keep a number of balls in the air. He also says it may not take all that much more time to communicate well. Has that been your experience?

Jim Strain: Yes, it has, Lee. As a matter of fact, we looked at the communication skills of a number of physicians in a hospital setting and found one who particularly impressed the patients. They thought he gave them a lot of information. Yet when we followed him, he took exactly five minutes to communicate what the patients thought was important information that really met their needs. So I think it is possible to become perceptive, to become aware of the patient's needs, and to communicate in a shorter time. That is where experience comes in.

Gus Swanson: To follow up on your observation about a student slowing down an office practice, in the state of Washington we asked physicians who took students into their practices what that really cost. Our data show that it costs between $25,000 and $35,000 a year for a site that will accommodate two students for a period of nine months. I think we have to take that into account; we really do have to reimburse such costs.

Bob Pantell: If you look at the national data, it has always been interesting to me that pediatricians see more patients than internists, and I think they actually see more patients than recently graduated family practitioners, although general practitioners in general see more patients than pediatricians. I wonder if there isn't something of a self-esteem crisis among pediatricians in terms of how valuable communicating with the family really is. It seems that pediatrics has always been a high-volume practice, and I think that the fact that we do not have many procedures is part of the problem. Internists can bill $35 for an office electrocardiogram. Pediatricians just do not have procedures that they can charge for, other than a few immunizations in a child's first year. This is a problem because most physicians bill for about one and one-half times what the actual office visit costs, but pediatricians have to depend on volume to cover their costs. So I am wondering if we can get pediatricians and parents as well to see that time spent in counseling and communication is time worth paying for.

Jim Strain: I think there will be some changes in the fee structure which will allow pediatricians to spend more time on psychosocial issues. Very frankly, this is an economic problem. Pediatricians do 95 percent of their work in offices with an overhead of 50 percent, so they have to see a large volume of patients to make a go of it. I think that most pediatricians would like very much to spend 30 to 45 minutes with a patient, and many do and are charging appropriately. But we are not dealing with an affluent group of people, we are dealing with young families. Most of the insurance companies do not pay for preventive health care and for outpatient health care services for children. If such policies could be changed, I think it would be a help.

Earl Schaefer: Some pediatricians have nurse practitioners or other professionals who can provide consultations.

Jim Strain: Our most recent study showed that 10 percent of pediatricians work with nurse practitioners, and some use them very well. Others are very uncomfortable with having nurse practitioners counseling patients because they want to be the only one communicating with parents. Then, too, there is an economic problem. The nurse has to generate a certain amount of income which, probably more than any other one thing, is a restrictive factor.

Andy Selig: Are there any studies which show that spending more time communicating with people — even though it may not be directly reimbursable — pays off further down the line in terms of fewer frantic phone calls? That kind of pay-off level is another way to think about the economics at work.

Jim Strain: I do not know whether there has been such a study, Andy. But I can say anecdotally that the more time you spend with a mother in the hospital in the immediate newborn period going over the things she might experience at home, the fewer phone calls you get.

PUBLIC POLICY TO PROMOTE BETTER COMMUNICATION

Lisbeth Bamberger Schorr

I am struck by how much consensus this Round Table has achieved regarding the importance of effective communication, interpersonal skills, and a more collaborative relationship between health care practitioners and children, parents, and families. We agree on the importance of effective communication. We agree that effective communication can be taught. And we agree that it can and should be practiced more widely. So the question becomes why aren't these things happening?

Structural Barriers

In these remarks, I want to concentrate on the structural barriers that prevent effective communication. These barriers are related to public policy, and many have been mentioned repeatedly during this Round Table. Judy Igoe's paper shows how fee-for-service payment arrangements reinforce the acute care model. Chuck Lewis has talked about the fact that health professionals can't get paid for talking to parents, even though talking to parents is an essential part of changing children's behavior. Earl Schaefer has addressed this same issue, contending that the involvement of the parents is essential but time spent eliciting that involvement is not reimbursed. Jim Strain has spoken about how the pressure to design pediatric training to meet service needs obstructs more training in ambulatory care which is so badly reimbursed, especially when it involves teaching. Bob Chamberlin has said that preventive services don't reach the children who need them the most; he has noted that most health practitioners — in fact most health institutions — aren't set up to respond to complex life situations which may require intervention from a variety of separate service agencies. So it becomes very clear that the way we pay for health services and the way we allocate our health resources make it very hard to achieve the goals on which participants in this Round Table agree.

Several points relevant to these issues were raised by the Select

Panel for the Promotion of Child Health with which I was involved. The Panel was established by Congress and spent two years holding hearings around the country to learn the concerns of people who attempt to provide good health services to children. We also looked at a very large proportion of the studies that were available in the literature. As a result, the Panel emphasized the importance of changing health care financing arrangements. We did this because the way health services are financed seemed to us to be the single most important determinant of how the health care system operates, of what services are available, of which professionals provide services, and of who will receive them and in what circumstances.

The Panel made several recommendations about financing. One of these recommendations was that the incentives in public and private third-party payment systems as they now operate have to be changed. Current incentives result in an allocation of physician time, distribution of physicians by specialty, and a manner of providing health services that collectively are unresponsive to a significant part of patient needs. One of the biggest obstacles to health care communication that the Panel identified is the bias in third-party reimbursement toward hospital-based, technologically oriented care. Physicians and other health providers are consistently paid more for using technological procedures than for examining and talking with patients. And that disparity is growing, not lessening. Between 1975 and 1978, reimbursements from Blue Cross in Washington, D.C., for the performance of technological procedures increased by more than 50 percent, although reimbursements for physicians' time with patients went up only 20 percent. Of course, our Panel wasn't the first to recognize this trend. For example, the American Association of Medical Colleges has also concluded that payment for professionals who spend time listening to, examining, and counseling patients is so inadequate that generalists must keep their interval of time with each patient to a minimum, and must use this time to perform procedures.

Since 1980, budget cutbacks at the federal and state levels have exacerbated this situation further. Individual health providers and health institutions, in order to simply stay solvent, must act in ways that create a still greater mismatch between what patients need and the services which are reimbursed. As Bob Chamberlin has pointed out, the children for whom counseling and anticipatory guidance have been found to be least important are the only ones likely to be able to get it; those children who need guidance and counseling are the least likely to get it. There are already reports of children being seen at a more severe stage of illness (and even of some children presenting with illnesses that doctors in this country haven't seen for quite some time), possibly because primary and general care have become less accessible over the last year.

Suggestions for Change: Building Coalitions

Having identified some of the problems that exist today, I would like to make some suggestions about what can be done. The first has to do with building coalitions and networks. I found Kelley MacDonald's story very significant and instructive. She spoke of a group of parents, organized around a disease or a handicapping condition, who were able to advocate not only for their own children, but who were also able to change what Medicaid covered for other children in their state. Furthermore, some of the changes that these parents were able to bring about in hospital practices were not limited to just one group of children. The changes also benefited children who had other conditions and diseases.

We have talked a lot at this Round Table about how categorical advocacy groups seem to be easier to form than more broadly based groups, and how the narrowly focused groups seem to have a lot of power. I believe that if the groups broaden their areas of concern and the targets on behalf of whom they advocate, they will become more, not less, effective. This is not to say that broadening parents' groups is easy. A team at Vanderbilt University, which is studying chronically ill children, brought together categorical advocacy groups to see if the groups felt they had enough in common to be able to take on some issues together. They found it very difficult, yet I think that's the kind of effort we have to keep attempting.

In addition, I think categorical parents' groups and concerned health professionals may find it both useful and profitable to join with groups which have a considerably larger umbrella. Examples of these larger groups are the Association for the Care of Children's Health (formerly the Association for the Care of Children in Hospitals), the Junior League (which has made child health one of its major emphases), and the Children's Defense Fund (which I think comes closest to trying to take on children's issues of all kinds). As categorical groups and professionals are able to connect with these broader groups, the resulting coalitions are likely to be increasingly effective in changing state and federal policies and financial incentives.

Suggestions for Change: Financial Incentives

It seems to me that there is one notable, hopeful note in current demands for cost-containment. These demands may act to upset the status quo in such a way that people who want to see changes in financing that go beyond cost-containment are more likely to be heard. These are needed in both public and private third-party payment programs. Revisions of payment schedules and payment methods which adequately reflect the value of counseling and other time-intensive aspects of primary care are needed, as are revisions to lessen inappropriate incentives for performing technical procedures. In addition, third-party payment programs should be changed to include various methods of paying for packages of services, such as lump-sum payments for specified services or for a specified period of time. Obstetricians have been utilizing such approaches for a long time, and some pediatricians are now also beginning to use them. Another reimbursement change that is needed is one which would offer equal incentives for training health professionals in ambulatory settings and in patient care settings. To bring about these kinds of reimbursement changes, coalitions of parents and professionals may not only have to go beyond disease categories, they may even have to go beyond age categories.

Related to the need for changes in financial incentives is the issue of paying for services which are not now reimbursed by third-party payers. This category of services includes counseling, anticipatory guidance, and other services which are difficult to define and standardize, and which are often seen as vulnerable to both provider and patient abuse. In addition, there is very little consensus about who should be providing these services. For example, can a lay health visitor provide a home health visit as well as a nurse? Many of these services are often best provided outside of health facilities. A lot of them have prevention as at least one of their purposes, and it is much more difficult to evaluate effectiveness when something other than curing is the purpose of the service. As if that weren't complicated enough, there is also very little consensus as to which of these services should be provided by or through the health system, rather than through schools, religious institutions, informal networks, or social agencies.

Given these factors, the Select Panel came to the conclusion that a new institution is needed that could systematically review some of these services and make recommendations to third-party payers regarding their coverage. If this institution, which the Panel called a Board on Health Services Standards, included enough prestigious and authoritative individuals, it might be able to make recommendations about which of these "soft" services should be widely included in third-party payment programs and in what circumstances.

Suggested Changes: Advocacy by Health Professionals

And now to my last point. It would be nice if the financial underpinnings for the kinds of services that we're talking about could be provided without parents and professionals having to take on the struggle for universal coverage of all health services for all children. However, national policy is moving toward letting market forces take over and distribute resources. At a recent meeting of the National Association of Children's Hospitals and Related Institutions, three leaders of medicine told the audience that health providers have to become entrepreneurs and businessmen. They said, in effect, "We've got to provide services that people are going to buy." There were fears expressed by many of the hospitals' administrators and trustees that they were going to have to orient their services to the people who could pay for them if they were going to stay open, and that they were going to have to turn their backs on children and families who don't have their own resources.

It seems to me that those who would leave the distribution of health services to market forces ignore the fact that society has a tremendous stake in the health status of children and pregnant women and in the kinds of health services they get. The "safety net" which is supposedly for those who "fall through the cracks" when the market forces take over (in the case of children Title V, Medicaid, and EPSDT) is being radically cut back in both benefits and beneficiaries. In addition, most states have never supported programs with patterns of care which promote the kind of continuity and follow-up that we have identified as essential. So those of us who understand the consequences of very vulnerable children being denied the full benefit of modern health care really have to be in the forefront of advocacy for better state and national policies. We must work to assure that every American child and family not only have access to but receive the full array of needed health and health-related services. Failing such a development, the good communication that this Round Table has been envisioning will be most unlikely to reach many of those who need it most urgently.

DISCUSSION

Bob Chamberlin: Lee, what is happening in regard to the National Board on Health Services Standards that your Select Panel suggested?

Lisbeth Schorr: Members of the Select Panel are discussing this idea in a variety of forms, but the closest that anyone from outside the

Panel has come to advocating something similar was in a recent *New England Journal of Medicine* article by David Rogers, the President of the Robert Wood Johnson Foundation. He reviewed the effects of Medicaid cuts and said that the cuts were being made in precisely the wrong areas. He said that instead of having state legislatures make these decisions, some sort of professional board should decide where cuts would do the least harm.

Chuck Lewis: As you probably know, some time in the next year, the Institute of Medicine will hold a conference which will be sponsored in part by the Johnson Foundation. It will examine standards of medical practice, and it may represent the last time for professionals to make a statement about the things that we think ought to be done and the sort of standards we as professionals want.

Lisbeth Schorr: The Panel suggested that one of the places where a Board on Health Services Standards might be located was, in fact, in the Institute of Medicine. We felt that the need for this kind of a mechanism is going to increase over time as the rate of knowledge increases, and considered it essential that the Board be established in a setting where its work could continue over time.

Gus Swanson: One comment on the matter of categorical advocacy groups: I think that the usual behavior of advocacy groups is to forget about everybody elses' needs and go after their own. For example, an Institute of Arthritis is about to be established at the National Institutes of Health, which is a prime example of the power of single issue groups in medicine.

Lisbeth Schorr: But of course it is also true that the combined efforts of all single issue groups have probably resulted in more funding for the National Institutes of Health than if the Institutes had never been organized along categorical lines. That is why I think models like the Children's Defense Fund, which goes into a community and tries to get the various parents' groups that are organized along categorical lines to work together, are valuable. The Fund has found that the groups often have a lot in common. For example, they have found that the parents of handicapped children face many of the same problems as the parents of children who belong to racial and economic minority groups.

Jon Ziarnik: While we are talking about coalitions for health funding, I am somewhat disturbed by some of the themes that keep running through our discussions. I am wondering if it is possible to talk about communication without putting so much emphasis on cost-containment. I guess I really am worried when we say, "We don't get paid to talk to people, we get paid for performing technological procedures." I understand that money is a concern — it has to be. But I guess I do not see it as the major reason for people to behave or not behave in a caring and compassionate way.

Kelley MacDonald: I just wanted to comment about how ironic I think it is to talk about how parents' groups should be advocating third-party billing for professionals when the parents' groups themselves have no billable hours.

Joy Penticuff: Aside from categorical groups in the community in which I live, there really isn't enough community awareness of the needs of all children. If you are a middle-class person, then your children and the children of all your neighbors go to pediatricians, and there is no big problem. You frankly are not really aware of the plight of many children in other neighborhoods.

Lisbeth Schorr: I think there are going to be more and more middle-class people who are going to lose their jobs and their health insurance, and who may not qualify for Medicaid. Then larger and larger numbers of American families are going to find out some things that are wrong with our system that they did not know anything about before.

I just want to make one more comment about the issue Jon raised. While the third-party payment plans make the distinction between communication (and other "soft" services) and medicine, I do not believe that they can be separated. However, I think it is important to identify which services are being systematically under-reimbursed. You really have to look at where the money is coming from and how financing decisions are made because otherwise what we are talking about becomes fanciful.

APPENDIX A

COMMUNICATION GUIDELINES

The Pediatric Round Table from which the following communication guidelines emerged included health and human services professionals (both in private practice and in teaching and administrative positions) as well as health consumers and parents with children with handicapping conditions. While participants recognized the importance of communications between health professionals, the importance of mass media communications regarding health, the importance of the technological aspects of communications research, and the important impact of health systems on child health, the Round Table could not effectively cover all these areas in depth in the limited time available (three days). Therefore, participants focused on interpersonal communications between health professionals, children, and families, and the following guidelines should be viewed in this light.

ASSUMPTIONS ON WHICH THE GUIDELINES ARE BASED

1. Sponsors of and participants in the Round Table have come to believe, on the basis of their own work and experience and the relevant work of others, that improved interpersonal communications can enhance child health status and family functioning.
2. The Round Table was intended to identify and disseminate information about specific mechanisms through which improved communications might be accomplished.

   Participants believe that the consequences of improved communications are measurable (although the Round Table was not set up to collect and review this evidence) and include the following: decreased suffering; decreased morbidity and mortality; lowered health costs; greater patient and family satisfaction; improved child and family functioning; increased health professional satisfaction and productivity; and improved coordination of services among health care providers.
3. Round Table participants believe that there are many ways in which improved communication leading to better child health

outcomes can be brought about. Some of the strategies for bringing about such improvements included the following:
   a. Explicit education of health professionals in communication skills should occur at every level of training. This includes taking interpersonal communication skills into account when screening and selecting applicants to health professional schools, and when providing continuing education and training at the postgraduate level. This training should be integrated with biomedical education; nurturing of health professionals should occur at every level of training and activity to enhance their capacity for supportive interpersonal interactions; and respected and valued mentors should be models of interpersonal communication skills.
   b. Financing and organization of health services delivery should permit and encourage the use of good interpersonal communication skills by not economically penalizing those who take the time necessary to practice these skills.
   c. There should be action by all persons involved (including parents, families, patients, self-help consumer groups, groups of concerned citizens, and professionals) to bring about desired changes in health institutions, in the allocation of resources, in health legislation, and in administration of health programs.
   d. Licensing and certification agencies and boards should expand their efforts to assess health professionals' competence in interpersonal communication skills.
4. Round Table participants recognize that while good health care is only one factor determining health status, it is a very important factor; participants furthermore agree that good communication is an essential component of high quality health services, rather than a goal which might compete with excellence in technical care.

GUIDELINES FOR MORE EFFECTIVE INTERPERSONAL COMMUNICATION TO IMPROVE CHILD HEALTH

General Guidelines

1. Effective interpersonal communication involves verbal and nonverbal communication and cognitive and affective exchanges. It is also interactive; that is, health professionals *and* patients/families must be involved if effective communication is to occur.
2. Good communication is enhanced by continuity in the provider-patient/family relationship.
3. Health professionals who care for children should use a systems-

oriented approach. That is, they should be aware that the cause and effect of what is observed, what is planned, and what is done go beyond the individual child to involve the child's family and community.

Guidelines for Improving Communications Between Providers and Children/Families

4. Health professionals should make an individualized, tailored response to each child and family, making an effort to understand and take into account the context of the child's health status, developmental stage, level of cognitive development, history, and family and social context (including family functioning, socioeconomic circumstances, belief system, culture, etc.).
5. To communicate effectively, the health professional should use appropriate language, and should be able to draw from a large repertoire of ways of responding to or engaging in exchanges with the child/family.
6. The health professional should be willing and able to elicit and respond to the child's/family's agenda and concerns for the encounter.
7. The health professional should understand a child's/family's values and then collaborate with the child/family in decisions regarding treatment, follow-up, and management; the professional should be willing and able to encourage child/family use of their own resources and coping skills; and the health professional should support the maximum level of child/family participation in decision-making that the child/family is willing to assume.
8. To bring about effective communication leading to better follow-up, more effective adherence to prescribed (agreed upon) regimen, etc., the health professional should be able to establish mutual trust, and make the child/family feel understood, respected, and included in both the diagnostic and treatment processes.
9. Health professionals should value their skills as educators, and should see this as central to their role as facilitators of child and family functioning in promoting health and coping with illness; professionals should be able to interact effectively with individuals who have different styles of learning and communicating.
10. Health professionals should encourage children/families to communicate their concerns, questions, dissatisfactions, etc., and should let the children/families know that they will respond to those concerns. In addition, all professionals concerned with

communications with children must recognize the social context of childhood, i.e., the basic cultural values and norms which influence the roles children play in any society, including what children are expected to say, when, and to whom.

Guidelines for Systems Changes

11. Although the family is the primary coordinator of child care, it is imperative that one qualified professional be identified to coordinate communication when a number of health professionals are involved in the care of a child; this person should be both powerful and influential within the health system, and should have continuity in his or her relationship with the child/family.

APPENDIX B

SELECTED COMMUNICATION EXAMPLES

The following descriptions are of programs, projects, or other efforts which are designed to enhance communication for child health. They have been selected from *Communications Examples for Child Health,** which was initially developed for use by participants attending the Round Table. Subsequently, the decision was made to publish the communication examples in hopes that interested professionals and laypersons might be able to adapt some portions of them for use in other clinics, hospitals, training programs, and communities.

While the communication examples provide a brief description of some innovative efforts underway across the United States, they were not developed in conjunction with the Communication Guidelines (Appendix A). As a result, there is not a perfect "fit" between the two. For example, some of the examples deal with communications be-

---

*To order complete set of *Communications Examples for Child Health,* see last page of this section for order form.

tween health professionals, an area which the Communication Guidelines did not address. The editors have not attempted to evaluate the effectiveness of the examples which follow, and wish to stress that the examples certainly do not represent the *only* communication efforts for child health underway in this country. The lack of time and space has unfortunately precluded the inclusion of many worthwhile projects and programs.

In an effort to make the communication examples useful for persons with a wide range of interests, they have been grouped into six categories. Selected examples from each category are as follows.

EDUCATIONAL/TRAINING PROGRAMS FOR PROFESSIONALS

Training in Conveying Distressful Information

Both residents and medical students at the University of Iowa's Hospitals and Clinics receive training which involves videotapes and which focuses on conveying distressful information to parents.

During residency training, students meet with simulated mothers who have been trained to act a part in one of three different situations. In the first situation, the resident must tell the "mother" that her newborn has Down's syndrome. In the second, the resident has to tell the "mother" that she is going to be reported for child abuse. And in the third situation, the resident talks with the "mother" of a multiply handicapped toddler; this session is less stressful because the "parent" already knows about the child's handicaps. The resident's performance during these sessions is videotaped, and the resident views the tapes with a staff member who offers constructive criticism when necessary.

Mark Wolraich, M.D., says that the approach, which has been in use for six years, is very popular with housestaff, and evaluation results have been good. To objectively determine the effects of the training, residents' performances were videotaped both at the beginning and end of training (using similar "problem" scenarios), and the videotapes were independently and blindly rated. The residents' skills and sensitivity were shown to significantly improve between the pre- and post-test simulations.

The University's staff realized that medical students also needed similar training, but faced the reality that the one-on-one approach used with residents was too time-consuming. Therefore, one year ago, a Micro Counseling Techniques Course was developed for medical students. In this course, a counseling psychology graduate student worked with a group of six medical students, teaching the students techniques of giving information to patients and ways of dealing with patients' affective responses. The students role played behaviors of an interviewer and a patient among themselves.

The effectiveness of this course for medical students is now being evaluated, and results should be available soon. Wolraich says that a problem which remains with the course is that the six-to-one ratio is still too high for most medical schools. Therefore, the project's staff have applied for a grant to fund the development of training videotapes which, it is hoped, could be used with larger groups.

For information, contact:
Mark Wolraich, M.D.
University Hospital School
University of Iowa
Iowa City, IA 52242

History Checklist and Interview Rating Scale

One approach to teaching medical students to effectively take a history and conduct an interview has been developed at the University of Arizona College of Medicine. There, nonphysicians have been trained as simulated parents who are interviewed by first, second, and third year medical students.

The "patient-instructors" use as much real history information as possible so that their training period is kept short. For example, a learning disabilities teacher may use the history of a child in her class and present the history as if talking about her own child. Or a nurse who has worked on a cancer ward may use a history of a child with leukemia.

A number of medical schools use simulated patients to teach history-taking and interviewing skills. What is unusual about the University of Arizona's approach is the use of a History Content Checklist and the Arizona Clinical Interview Rating Scale, both of which were developed for the program. In addition, the interviews are conducted without the necessity of a physician observer.

Following an interview, the simulated parent and medical student switch roles, and the patient-instructor goes over both forms with the students. The patient-instructor reviews the History Content Checklist, telling the medical students what items they neglected to ask, suggesting ways they could have gotten the desired information, and giving the student a history content score.

Then the patient-instructor reviews the Arizona Clinical Interview Rating Scale with the student. This scale contains 14 items, including such things as questioning skills, documentation of information, eye contact, and so on. The instructor goes through each item, commenting, "You did well here," or, "You could improve here. Let me give you an example of how you could have done it better." The students also get a performance score, which can run from poor through excellent, on this scale.

The program with simulated parents as patient-instructors utilizing the two forms has been underway in Arizona for seven years. One of the program's developers says that thousands of interviews have been given, and that the medical students are very enthusiastic about the approach. However, Paula Stillman, M.D., notes that this approach was not as enthusiastically received when it was used for two years with pediatric house officers. She says, "The house officers didn't like being evaluated very well. I think how they feel about this approach depends on how the program director presents it," because internal medicine and family practice housestaff are currently using it at the University without objection.

Stillman says that the program has been used with practicing physicians very successfully. This is probably because the physicians themselves have requested the training (through continuing medical education).

Considerable evaluation of the Arizona approach has been conducted. For example, research showed that students' scores on the Clinical Interview Rating Scale rose following a training interview, and that the greatest amount of learning (as measured by improved scores on the scale) occurred during the first interview. When a group of students were followed over time, there was found to be no drop in skill levels after 12 months.

Stillman says that the program, which began with a grant, is currently funded by the state as part of the medical school curriculum. She notes that it is not an expensive approach. For example, it could be started with only three patient-instructors.

For additional information, or to obtain the History Content Checklist and the Arizona Clinical Interview Rating Scale, contact:

Paula L. Stillman, M.D.
Associate Dean
University of Massachusetts
Medical School
55 Lake Avenue North
Worcester, MA 01605

PROGRAMS TO TEACH PARENTS COMMUNICATION SKILLS
Perinatal Coaching Program

A program to train parents to understand, handle, and interact effectively with their newborn child is the Perinatal Coaching Program. It trains lay parents to be "coaches" for new parents, beginning while the baby is still in the hospital and continuing for several weeks after the baby is discharged.

The perinatal period was selected for this preventive program because it is an ideal time to promote parent-child communication, and because it is during this period that first-time parents are most eager to learn about their infant. The program's developers felt that it would be most effective if it were both hospital- and office-based (as opposed to being based simply in one of those settings) because it would then span the period immediately after birth and following discharge from the hospital. The Perinatal Coaching Program expands what is most commonly taught to parents about their baby, with an emphasis on how the parents can learn to be sensitive to the behavior and communication.

New parents are usually approached first in the hospital by the child's physician, who tells the parents that a perinatal coach is available to help them learn about babies and how to communicate with them. In almost all cases, the parents are eager to have this assistance.

The hospital nurses are alerted that the parents will be visited by the coach, who usually arrives that evening to begin the first of four 60- to 90-minute sessions. The coach uses a book of pictures specially developed for this training in addition to the newborn to demonstrate how to communicate with the baby. The thrust of this first session is to build a positive interaction between parents and child.

The remaining three sessions involve practice and demonstration of these skills. However, the fourth session differs from the others in that it is conducted in the family's home several days after discharge of the baby from the hospital. Holding the final coaching session some time after discharge provides positive reinforcement for the parents, and permits the coach to see if the family is coping adequately or if the parents may need assistance from a professional within the community.

The volunteer coaches receive special training so that they will be effective as trainers. The training takes about six hours (usually in three two-hour sessions) and covers infants' sensory abilities, states of consciousness, and basic communication skills, as well as a baby's unique qualities as an individual. Training materials for coaches are distributed without charge by Gerber Products Company, and include a checklist, written materials, and a slide-tape. Two training videotapes are available for a small fee. The coaches learn that modeling, demonstration, observation, positive feedback, and practice are all critical elements if perinatal coaching is to be effective.

The major expense of the program is for the salary of the trainer/

coordinator, usually a hospital- or office-based professional. The coordinator recruits parents to be coaches, maintains a follow-up system with community services for those parents who need them, and generally sees that close communication is maintained between hospital and office or clinic.

For more information about the program, contact:
>   Ray E. Helfer, M.D.
>   Department of Pediatrics and Human Development
>   College of Human Medicine
>   B 240 Life Science Building
>   Michigan State University
>   East Lansing, MI 48824
>   (517) 353-4583

Free materials for training coaches are available from:
>   Perinatal Coaching Kit Part I
>   Gerber Products Company
>   Marketing Division
>   445 State Street
>   Fremont, MI 49421

PROGRAMS FOR FAMILIES WITH CHRONICALLY ILL OR HANDICAPPED CHILDREN

Coalition of Advocacy Groups

The Federation for Children with Special Needs is a coalition of 10 statewide organizations developed by parents who have children with a wide range of special problems such as mental retardation, spina bifida, learning disabilities, and cardiac problems. One project of the Federation seeks to provide forums to involve both parents and health professionals.

Coordinator of a Parent-Professional Collaboration on Medical Issues Project, Betsy Anderson, says that the project developed because most health settings — especially private health settings — typically had little parent involvement. Anderson says, "It is very rare for any of the parents to be asked for feedback about the services their child was getting. We felt that as 'experienced' parents, so to speak, we had a lot of good information to share, but there was no structured or obvious way we could give input to professionals."

The Federation therefore sought and received a Department of Education grant to help facilitate communication between parents and professionals. Project staff members, all who have special needs children, began by contacting medical settings and saying that they were parents who would like to talk with the health professionals. As

Anderson notes, "They seemed surprised. In fact, at first they thought we wanted *them* to talk to *us*."

Another example of difficulties the project's staff encountered when they first attempted to bring parents and professionals together involved an effort to talk with pediatric residents. Anderson says, "We wanted to talk with them because they're often the ones parents see when their child is hospitalized. So we called a house officer at a hospital and asked if we could come out to speak with the residents. He was very enthusiastic at first, but then he called back and said they wanted to have the residents talk to the psychiatry department before we came, to see how the residents felt about parents."

Now, in its second year of a three-year grant, the project's staff and interested professionals go to hospital departments and other tertiary care settings to talk with health teams or with groups of nurses, social services professionals, etc. Anderson says, "While feelings of course underlie what we talk about, feelings aren't a topic that some groups (for example, surgeons) are comfortable discussing. So we try to develop a topic with an involved professional that will be relevant and interesting."

An example of one such topic is a presentation prepared for the staff of a hospital's radiology department. According to Anderson, the presentation was made by two parents, one who has a child who has to frequently undergo painful tests within the department, and one who has an autistic child. "The mother of the autistic child has devised unique ways to prepare her child for testing that makes it less traumatic, and we thought that the professionals who see other children whose understanding is limited or very different might want to know the techniques this mother has developed."

Anderson says that the group does not simply "go in and lecture." Instead, the parents (or parent-professional team depending on the presentation) speak briefly, and then encourage discussion. She says that one problem is getting enough time to do this effectively: "One 45-minute session really isn't enough, but often it's all that's available."

In addition to conducting such sessions for professionals, the project staff holds discussion and training sessions for parents. On one level, the sessions provide information to parents about their rights, resources, and so on. On another level, the staff trains parents to speak to and work with professionals. For example, topics include such things as parents' role in decision-making in the management of medical care, and communicating and information-sharing in medical settings. Whenever possible, these parent groups also include professionals so that different views can be shared.

The project has an advisory board which includes both parents and professionals. The professionals are especially valuable, according to Anderson, in devising strategies which will make other professionals *want* to learn from and be involved with parents.

For additional information, contact:
>Betsy Anderson or
Nora Wells
Federation for Children with Special Needs
312 Stuart Street
Boston, MA 02116
(617) 482-2915

SCHOOL-BASED PROGRAMS

Project Health P.A.C.T.

A unique consumer health education program teaches children from preschool age through high school to participate in their health care visits and to work collaboratively with health professionals to solve problems and develop appropriate plans of care. Project Health P.A.C.T. (Participatory and Assertive Consumer Training) is an award-winning program developed at the University of Colorado School of Nursing's School Health Programs. P.A.C.T. teaches children to communicate effectively with health professionals through the use of five health consumer rules or behaviors. These are: (1) talk with the health professional and share information about yourself; (2) listen and learn about new ways to take care of yourself; (3) ask questions; (4) decide what to do with help from the health professional; and (5) do follow through on plans that have been jointly decided upon.

Children are usually first introduced to the P.A.C.T. rules in their school classrooms. In this environment, various teaching strategies are used to establish the new consumer behaviors. The teacher, school nurse, and the P.A.C.T. materials model ways that the children can assertively but politely ask questions of health professionals. Next, children practice what they have learned in the school health office, where school nurses help refine and shape the children's new consumer skills by providing positive feedback for appropriate responses. Finally, having learned and practiced their newly acquired skills, the children are ready to implement their role as health consumers in other community health settings.

The approach for teaching P.A.C.T. is based on the observational learning theory. Teaching methods include role modeling and imitation, shaping (role playing), and positive reinforcement.

The models on which P.A.C.T.'s materials and approaches were designed take into account the developmental characteristics of children at different ages. For children in preschool through grade two, a cognitive-developmental model is used. Based on Piaget's theories, this model encourages children to learn by labeling and classifying. The professional presenting the program plays a major role in helping the children learn and verbalize. An exploratory model is used for children from grades three through six; they are given hands-on experience in the school clinic, and more practice in modeling desired communication skills. A group process model is used for children in junior and senior high; adolescents learn by experiencing the reactions of their peers and by problem-solving with them. High school students use a health text and are taught such self-help skills as how to take their own blood pressure. In addition, adolescents learn about the developmental stages of younger children so that they can — with supervision — help younger students be participatory health consumers.

Age-appropriate materials developed to assist children learn this new consumer role include bright and interesting orientation coloring books and comic books, student workbooks with accompanying teacher manuals, health history books to be filled out by the children with assistance from parents, as well as filmstrips/slide tape presentations demonstrating the participatory assertive consumer role. For example, preschoolers through second graders use a coloring book which features a teddy bear-like creature called "Kip." Third graders through fourth graders use a "Zy-Exelon" comic book, which features a child from the planet "Megalos." "Zy-Exelon" is green, has three eyes, and a pedestal instead of feet; an earth child teaches him how to communicate effectively with health professionals. Children in fifth and sixth grade use the "Mighty Health Team" comic book, which includes characters that resemble Wonder Woman, Superman, and so on. For junior high students, there is a "Responsible You" activity book.

P.A.C.T. does not always have to be initiated at school. A physician or nurse's office might be the central training site for P.A.C.T. In these instances the organizer is advised to send the parent and the child a letter explaining how the program encourages children to become more involved during their health visit. P.A.C.T. materials may also be sent in advance so that parent and child can become acquainted with the new approach and have time to think up questions to ask.

The program's developers stress that a community-wide effort is necessary if P.A.C.T. is to be effective. They recommend that persons introducing the program to a community bring together parents and representatives of all the major health providers' groups to discuss P.A.C.T. in advance. This helps ensure that health providers and parents will be supportive when children attempt to ask questions and model an assertive health consumer role following their practice in school.

Evaluation of P.A.C.T. was undertaken with 278 students in eight fifth grade classes in three different Colorado school districts. In all three districts, the children using the program's materials and receiving its lectures and other activities had more gains in cognitive and affective areas than children who had simply viewed traditional health films, as well as more gains than children who received P.A.C.T.'s lectures but none of the program's materials. P.A.C.T.'s developers say that parents are pleased with the changes they see in their children following the program, for the children ask more questions, want to know more about good health habits and simple first aid, and accept more responsibility for their own health and health visits.

A nationwide evaluation of Project Health P.A.C.T. is scheduled to begin this fall with funding from the federal government.

Because it is easier to teach children cognitive skills than social skills, workshops are run each summer at the University of Colorado School of Nursing to help professionals use the P.A.C.T. approach. In these workshops, professionals learn not only how to present materials, but also how to help children role model the P.A.C.T. approach.

For additional information, contact:
> Judith B. Igoe, R.N., M.S.
> School of Nursing
> University of Colorado Health Sciences Center
> 4200 East Ninth Avenue, C-287
> Denver, CO 80262
> (303) 394-7435

PROGRAMS FOR HOSPITALIZED CHILDREN AND THEIR FAMILIES

Teaching Children to Cope with Cancer Procedures

A research study which began in Oklahoma and will be continued in Los Angeles has resulted in a program which teaches children with cancer to cope with painful medical procedures. This kind of effort is necessary because children with cancer routinely have to endure many such procedures as spinal taps and bone marrow aspirations. Frequently the children are terrified, and have to be physically restrained while the procedures are conducted.

In an attempt to give children some ways to cope with the fear and pain of the procedures, a five-part intervention program was begun at Children's Hospital at the University of Oklahoma Health Sciences Center. "Filmed modeling" was the first component in the intervention program. Children and their parents saw a film of another child successfully cope with the medical procedures. The child on the film talks about her thoughts and feelings (including, "I'm scared, but I can handle it"). The film also tells children why the procedure has to be done and what it's about.

Following the film, professionals in the Psychosocial Program taught the children relaxation and breathing exercises. These exercises helped to distract and relax the children while they were undergoing the procedures.

Third, the children were offered trophies if they stayed still during the procedures and did their breathing exercises. The little trophies, complete with their name, were very popular with elementary school-age children, according to Susan Jay, Ph.D., a psychologist who helped implement the program. (Jay says she never denied a child a trophy even if they struggled during a procedure. However, sometimes parents would withhold the trophy saying, "Let's see if you can do better next time.")

Fourth, the children were taught to use imagery and fantasy. Jay says this varied with the child, but that children with a special "superhero," for example, might be asked to pretend that they were Superman's assistant, and that Superman had asked them to undergo the medical tests as part of a special mission.

Finally, the children were given three behavioral rehearsals. They were given a doll and actual medical materials, and allowed to do a bone marrow and spinal tap on the doll. They next pretended that they were the doctor and did a "tap" as the professional pretended to be the child and modeled desired coping behavior ("I'm scared now, so I will practice my breathing exercises"). When these two rehearsals had been completed, the children themselves pretended to undergo the procedure while the professional coached them.

All these steps in the program, from viewing the film through behavioral rehearsals, were taken the morning of the procedure, after which the children were "pretty well psyched up for the procedure" according to Jay. The professional would then accompany the child and parents as the actual procedure was done, helping and coaching the child throughout. The preparation of children was usually conducted the day of the procedure, Jay says, because some children were too young to remember for long what they had learned, and others didn't want to think about what lay ahead until they had to. If an older child had been a real problem during previous procedures, the training might be given in advance of a procedure, and parents would then be asked to practice the relaxation and breathing exercises with the child at home.

Children with cancer generally receive a bone marrow aspiration or spinal tap every two to three months, depending on their condition and on the health facility involved. Prior to each subsequent tap, the child would be given a "booster session" under this program. The film, exercises, and rehearsals were all reviewed again unless the child wished to skip part of the preparation.

The research conducted in conjunction with this program involved having an observer measure the child's distress level during the procedure on an observation scale developed by Jay; having the child rate the amount of pain on a "pain thermometer"; having a nurse rate the child's anxiety level; and measuring the child's heart rate. (Future research, which will be carried out at Children's Hospital in Los Angeles will also measure children's pulse rate, blood pressure, and sweat.)

The research from the Oklahoma pilot study was conducted with 10 children, and showed that nine of the children had a decrease in distress levels of at least 40 to 50 percent or more. (The tenth child's distress level dropped after a second orientation with the program.) The study also showed that the distress level of the children increased somewhat the second time a procedure was performed — although the level was not as high as it had been on the baseline.

A three-year study based on pilot results was recently funded by the National Cancer Institute and will be carried out at Children's Hospital in Los Angeles. Emphasis in the research project will be on comparing the techniques used in this program to the use of tranquilizing sedatives to calm children for painful spinal and bone marrow taps as well as a control condition.

Jay says that there was no opposition to the program from the parents in Oklahoma. "If it will help, parents of these children are willing to try almost anything," she says. She also says that physicians were very supportive once they had seen the film and had the program's psychosocial approach described to them. Funding was not a major problem, for the program and research were carried out very inexpensively. The greatest expense was for production of the film, which was donated by a parents' group called the Oklahoma Pediatric Cancer Association, and by the Department of Psychiatry at the University.

Jay says that the only real problem encountered involved a few children (two of 12) whose anxiety levels were raised by viewing the film and practicing the coping techniques. According to Jay, "Like adults, some kids have different coping styles, and may do better going into a procedure with no advanced information. This is something we hope to learn to predict in the future."

For additional information, contact:

>Susan Jay, Ph.D.
>Psychosocial Program
>Hematology-Oncology
>Children's Hospital
>4650 Sunset Boulevard
>Los Angeles, CA 90054
>(213) 660-2450, ext. 2392

PROGRAMS FOR PROFESSIONALS IN PRACTICE

Group Well Child Care

The use of groups in well child visits, which may be one way to enhance communication and improve child health, has been studied in Salt Lake City. There eight health professionals (four pediatricians, three family physicians, and one family nurse practitioner) saw groups of four to six mother-infant pairs in an effort to determine whether group well child visits are as effective and efficient as traditional, individualized visits. The practice settings represented were a large multi-specialty group, a health maintenance organization, a practice group, and a two-man partnership. Each experimental visit consisted of a 45-minute group discussion followed by brief individual physical examinations of the babies.

When the experimental and control groups were compared, group sessions were found to be as efficient as traditional well child visits. Babies in the groups received an average of 52 minutes of shared professional time (versus 16 minutes per individual visit). In addition, mothers in the groups were found to more regularly attend the well child visits although they paid the same full fee as for individual visits. Mothers in the groups asked more direct questions, and physicians working with the groups offered significantly more explanations. The mothers, who asked fewer questions of the physicians or nurses between visits, seemed to take more initiative during the visits, reassured one another by sharing experiences, and better used the professional as an information resource. Less time was found to be spent in the groups discussing the physical aspects of caring for a young child, while more time was spent discussing personal issues in the daily care of the baby. (Questions included family stress, the father's role in child rearing, sibling reactions to the new baby, and maternal depression.)

All but one of the mothers in the groups who were interviewed at the end of the study stated that they preferred the group method. They said they felt reassured by seeing the range of normal development displayed by the babies, by sharing common experiences, and by the questions which other mothers asked.

The professionals also liked the group approach. Six of the eight providers have said that they plan to continue their groups and/or form other groups. Sponsors of the study have speculated that the group well child visits have a number of advantages for health professionals. For example, approximately 40 percent of pediatricians' time is spent in well child care — a reality which, it can be seen, could rapidly lead to a sense of repetitiveness or even boredom. The group visit approach could help relieve this sameness in practice.

Problems with the group well child visit approach included the lack of space for group meetings in most medical practices, and the difficulty in scheduling a number of mother-infant pairs at the same time (especially as the babies got older and many mothers went back to work). In addition, the study's developers note that the mothers involved were entirely white and middle class. How such an approach would work with different ethnic or lower socioeconomic groups is unknown.

For additional information, contact:
>Lucy Osborn, M.D.
>Department of Pediatrics, #12-311
>University of California at Los Angeles
>Center for Health Sciences
>Los Angeles, CA 90024
>(213) 825-9346

BIBLIOGRAPHY

Aarons A, Hawes H: *Child to Child.* London and Basingstoke, MacMillan Press Ltd, 1979, p 104

Adams D: Children's response to a belt restraint program. *Pediatr Nurs* 1982; 8:28

Allen JM: Influencing school-age children's concept of hospitalization. *Pediatr Nurs* 1978; 8:28

An overview of the general professional education of the physician and college preparation for medicine and some questions that should be addressed. Washington, DC, Association of American Medical Colleges, 1982

Apley J: Listening and talking to patients V: communicating with children. *Br Med J* 1980; 281:1116-1117

Bain DJG: The content of physician/patient communication in family practice. *J Fam Pract* 1979; 8:745

Bandura A, Menlove, FL: Factors determining vicarious extinction of avoidance behavior through symbolic modeling. *J Personality & Socl Psychol* 1968; 8:99-108

Beck GR, Edgar E, Kenowitz L, Sulzbacher S, Lovitt TC, Zweibel S: The physician-educator team: let's make it work. *J. School Health* 1978; 48:79-83

Belsky MS, Gross L: *How to Choose and Use Your Doctor.* Greenwich, CT, Fawcett Crest Book, 1975

Berg JK, Garrard J: Psychosocial support in residency training programs. *J Med Educ* 1980; 55:851

Beuf A: *Biting Off the Bracelet: A Study of Children in Hospitals.* Philadelphia, PA, University of Pennsylvania Press, 1979

Bibace R, Walsh M: Development of children's concepts of illness. *Pediatrics* 1980; 66:912

Brent DA: The residency as a developmental process. *J Med Educ* 1981; 56:417

Brown, R: Introduction. In *Talking to Children — Language Input and Acquisition.* Edited by Snow CE, Ferguson CA. Cambridge University Press, 1977

Bryan E, Berg B, Thunder SK, Warden MG: The primary care physician as a member of the educational team. *J School Health* 1978; 48(8):465-466

Casey PH, Whitt JK: Effect of the pediatrician on the mother-infant relationship. *Pediatrics* 1980; 65:815-820

Chamberlin RW: Management of preschool behavior problems. *Pediatr Clin of North Am* 1974; 21:33-47

Chamberlin R, Szumowski E, Zastowny T: An evaluation of efforts to educate mothers about child development in pediatric office practices. *Amer J Public Health* 1979; 69:875-885

Chamberlin R, Olds D, Dawson P (editors). *Conference exploring the use of home visitors to improve the delivery of preventive services to mothers with young children.* Privately printed, 1981 (Department of Pediatrics, Attention Dr. R. Hoekelman, University of Rochester Medical Center, Rochester, NY 14642)

Charges to working groups on the essential knowledge, fundamental skills, and personal qualities, values, and attitudes that should comprise the general professional education of the physician and college preparation for medicine. Washington, DC, Association of American Medical Colleges, 1982

Collins M: *Communication in Health Care.* St Louis, CV Mosby, 1977

Cummins RO, Smith RW, Inui TS: Communication failure in primary care. *JAMA* 1980; 243(16):1650-1652

Duff RS, Rowe DS, Anderson FP: Patient care and student learning in a pediatric clinic. *Pediatrics* 1972; 50:839-852

Duke PM: The role of the pediatrician in the adolescent's school. *Pediatr Clin of North Am* 1980; 27(1):163-171

Dunlop D, Higgins L, Ling N: Crisis intervention in basic nursing education. *J Nurs Educ* 1978; 17:37-41

Eland JM: *Minimizing the hurt.* Paper presented at the 17th Annual Conference of the Association for the Care of Children's Health, Seattle, WA, June 2-5, 1982

Fagin CM, Nusbaum JG: Parental visiting privileges in pediatric units: a survey. *J Nurs Admin* 1978; 7:24-27

Farrell M, Haley M, Magnasco J: Teaching interpersonal skills. *Nursing Outlook* 1977; 25:322-325

Feinberg L: Panel to seek basic shift in "brutal" medical school curriculum. *Washington Post,* October 19, 1982, p 2

Gortner SR: Strategies for survival in the practice world. *Am J Nurs* 1977; 77:618-619

Gots R, Kaufman A: *The People's Hospital Book.* New York, Crown Publishers, 1978

Greenberg S: *The Quality of Mercy: A Report on the Critical Condition of Hospitals and Medical Care in America.* New York, Atheneum, 1971

Gutelius M, Kirsch A, MacDonald S et al: Promising results from a cognitive stimulation program in infancy. *Clin Pediatr* 1972; 11:585-593

Hovland CI, Weiss W: The influence of source credibility on communication effectiveness. *Public Opinion Quarterly* 1951; 15:635-650

Infante MS (ed): *Crisis Theory: A Framework for Nursing Practice.* Keston, VA, Reston Publishing (a Prentice-Hall Company), 1982

Jensen PS: The doctor-patient relationship: headed for impasse or improvement? *Annals of Int Med* 1981; 95:769-771

Kahn GS, Cohen B, Jason H: The teaching of interpersonal skills in U.S. medical schools. *J Med Educ* 1979; 54:29-35

Kalisch B: An experiment in the development of empathy in nursing students. *Nurs Res* 1971; 20:202-211

Korsch BM: Practical techniques of observing interviewing and advising parents in pediatric practice as demonstrated in an attitude study project. *Pediatrics* 1956; 18(3):467-490

Korsch BM, Freemon B, Negrete VF: Practical implications of doctor-patient interaction and analysis for pediatric practice. *Amer J Disabled Child* 1971; 12:110

Korsch BM, Gozzi EK, Francis V: Gaps in doctor-patient commucation. 1. doctor-patient interaction and patient satisfaction. *Pediatrics* 1968; 42(5):855-871

Korsch BM, Negrete VF: Doctor-patient communication. *Scientific American,* August 1972; 227:66-74

Kushner T: Doctor-patient relationships in general practice: a different model. *J Med Ethics* 1981; 7:128-131

Leopold E: Whom do we reach? A study of health care utilization. *Pediatrics* 1978; 53:341-348

Levin A: *Talk Back to Your Doctor.* New York, Doubleday & Co, 1975

Levinson DJ, Darrow CN, Klein EB et al: *Seasons of a Man's Life.* New York, Random House, 1978

Ley P: Towards better doctor-patient communication. In *Communication Between Doctors and Patients.* Edited by Bennett AE. London, Nuffield Provincial Hospitals, 1976

Mathews D: The non-compliant patient. *Primary Care* 1975; 2:289

Mechanic D: The influence of mothers on their children's health attitudes and behavior. *Pediatrics* 1964; 33:444

Moss JR: Helping young children cope with the physical examination. *Pediatr Nurs* 1981; 7(2):17

Mumford E: *Interns: From Students to Physicians.* Cambridge, MA, Harvard University Press, 1970

Orem DE: *Nursing: Concepts of Practice* (2nd ed). New York, McGraw-Hill, 1980

Osborn, LM: Group well-child care: An option for today's children. *Pediatric Nursing* 1982; 36:306-308

Perrin EC, Gerrity PS: There's a demon in your belly: children's understanding of concepts regarding illness. *Pediatrics* 1981; 67:841

Physician's Desk Reference. Medical Economics Co., Oradell, NJ, 1983

Piaget J, Innhelder B: *The Psychology of the Child.* New York, Basic Books, 1969

Pittman PR: Videotaping: a technique for teaching basic communication skills. *Nurse Educator* 1977; 2:16

Project Health PACT Program. *Assertive health consumer questionnaire.* Denver, CO, School Health Programs, University of Colorado Health Sciences Center, 1980

Reisinger K, Bires J: Anticipatory guidance in pediatric practice. *Pediatrics* 1980; 66:889-892

Rimstidt NS: *Parent survey: child health care communications.* Author: 516 Hamilton Court, Bloomington, Indiana 47401, July 1982

Rimstidt NS: *Speak Up for Your Child's Health.* Bloomington, IN, Program Prepare, Developmental Training Center, Indiana University, March 1981

Rinzler, CA: Shape up, doc! *Health* 1982; 14:9-55

Rogers DE, Blendon RJ, Moloney TW: Who needs Medicaid? *N Engl J Med* 1982; 307(1):13-18

Rogers K: The case against routine visits. In *Controversies in Child Health and Pediatrics.* Edited by Smith D, Hokelman R. New York, McGraw-Hill, 1980

Rosenberg SG: Patient education: an educator's view. In *Compliance with Therapeutic and Preventive Regimes.* Edited by Sackett DL, Haynes RB. Baltimore, MD, Johns Hopkins University Press, 1976, p 95

Schaefer ES: Professional support for family care of children. In *Maternal and Child Health Practices: Problems, Resources, and Methods of Delivery* (2nd ed). Edited by Wallace HM, Gold EM, Oglesby AC. New York, John Wiley & Sons, 1982, pp 433-446

Schaefer ES, Edgerton M: Parent and child correlates of parental modernity. In *Parental Belief Systems.* Edited by Sigel IE. New

York, Lawrence Erlbaum, in press, 1983

Select panel for the promotion of child health. *Better Health for our Children: A National Strategy.* US Department of Health and Human Services, Government Printing Office, 1981

Siegel B, Donnelly JC: Enriching personal and professional development: the experience of a support group for interns. *J Med Educ* 1978; 53:908

Silver G: *Child Health: America's Future.* Germantown, MD, Aspen Systems Corporation, 1973

Skipper JK, Leonard RC: Children, stress, and hospitalization: a field experiment. *J Health & Soc Behav* 1968; 9:275

Starfield B, Barkowf S: Physicians' recognition of complaints made by parents about their children's health. *Pediatrics* 1969; 43:168-172

Stine O: Content and method of health supervision by physicians in child health conferences in Baltimore. *Amer J Public Health* 1962; 52:1858-1865

Strahilevitz A, Yunker R, Pichanick AM et al: Initiating support groups for pediatric houseofficers. *Clin Pediatr* 1982; 21:529

Szasz TS, Hollender MH: Concepts of the doctor-patient relationship. *Arch Intern Med* 1956; 97:586-588

Valko RJ, Clayton PJ: Depression in the internship. *J Disorders of the Nervous System* 1975; 36:26

Visintainer MA, Wolfer JA: Psychological preparation for surgical pediatric patients: the effects on children's and parents' stress responses and adjustment. *Pediatrics* 1975; 56(2): 187-202

Vorhaus MG: *The Changing Patient-Doctor Relationship.* New York, Horizon Press, 1957

Walsh S: Parents of asthmatic kids (PAK): a successful parent support group. *Pediatr Nurs* 1981; 7(3):28

Werner ER, Adler R, Robinson R, Korsch BM: Attitudes and interpersonal skills during pediatric internship. *Pediatrics* 1979; 63:491

Wold S: *School Nursing: A Framework for Practice.* St Louis, MO, CV Mosby, 1981

Wolfer JA, Visintainer MA: Prehospital psychological preparation for tonsillectomy patients: effects on children's and parents' adjustment. *Pediatrics* 1979; 64(5):646-655

Wynn M, Wynn A: *Prevention of Handicaps and the Health of Women.* London, Rutledge & Kegan, 1979

Yarrow L: Aliza: weeks of crisis. *Parents* 1982; 56:66-67

Zaborenko RN, Zaborenko LM: *The Doctor Tree.* Pittsburgh, PA, University of Pittsburgh Press, 1978

Fold 2 along solid line. Moisten gum and seal.

ORDER FORM

Please send me:

Book No.	Qty.	Title	Price	Total
119		Communication Examples	$4.00	

Other Titles in the Pediatric ROUND TABLE SERIES

111		copies of PRT #6 **BIRTH, INTERACTION AND ATTACHMENT**	$6.00	
112		copies of PRT #5 **INFANTS AT RISK**	$6.00	
113		copies of PRT #4 **THE COMMUNICATION GAME**	$6.00	
114		copies of PRT #3 **LEARNING THROUGH PLAY**	$6.00	
115		copies of PRT #2 **SOCIAL RESPONSIVENESS OF INFANTS**	$6.00	
116		copies of PRT #1 **MATERNAL ATTACHMENT AND MOTHERING DISORDERS**	$6.00	
117		copies of PRT #7 **MINIMIZING HIGH-RISK PARENTING**	$6.00	
118		copies of PRT #8 **CHILD HEALTH CARE COMMUNICATIONS**	$6.00	

Fold 1 along solid line.

	Plus Postage & Handling	$ 1.00
TOTAL:	Please find a check or money order (made payable to Johnson & Johnson Baby Products Co.) for:	$ _____
SPECIAL OFFER:		
☐	Please send complete set (8 books plus Examples) only $45.00 plus $3.00 postage and handling	$ _____

Please allow 4-6 weeks for delivery.

8 Last Name 22   23 First Name 37

42 Institution/Hospital 63

64 Street Address 85

86 City 103   104 105 State   106 Zip Code 110

Offer valid only in U.S.A.

| NO POSTAGE |
| NECESSARY |
| IF MAILED |
| IN THE |
| UNITED STATES |

BUSINESS REPLY MAIL
FIRST CLASS   PERMIT NO. 30   SOMERVILLE, NJ

POSTAGE WILL BE PAID BY ADDRESSEE

Johnson & Johnson

BABY PRODUCTS COMPANY
P.O. BOX 836
SOMERVILLE, N.J. 08876